To Judy, Nancy and harry
whose father taught
me about vacances.

Louis Cooper
11/16/71

Vaccines and Viruses

Also by Nancy Rosenberg

THE STORY OF MODERN MEDICINE
(with Dr. Lawrence Rosenberg)

NEW PARTS FOR PEOPLE
(with Reuven K. Snyderman, M.D.)

VACCINES AND VIRUSES

NANCY ROSENBERG and
LOUIS Z. COOPER, M.D.

A W. W. NORTON BOOK
Published by
GROSSET & DUNLAP, INC.
New York

Table of Contents

Acknowledgments

During the winter of 1969, in the Nigerian town of Lassa, an American missionary nurse fell seriously ill. She was dead within three days, of a strange disease that no one could identify. When a second nurse died the same way, an investigation was made. It revealed that Lassa fever was a brand-new disease, caused by a virus that had never been seen before.

New viruses are always turning up this way, and new and improved vaccines are constantly being developed. To make this book as accurate and up to date as possible, we consulted a number of the people currently involved in this work. Our thanks go to all of them for taking the time and the trouble to help us.

The late Dr. Wendell M. Stanley sent us a copy of his Nobel Lecture on the isolation and properties of the tobacco mosaic virus and an electron micrograph of the virus itself. Dr. D. A. Henderson reviewed for us the current status of smallpox as a world health problem.

During a fascinating visit to the Harvard laboratory of Dr. John F. Enders, we learned firsthand about the breakthroughs that led to the conquest of measles and polio. Further recollections of the early days in the development of the polio vaccine came from Dr. Alex J. Steigman.

For descriptions of the early trials of the measles vaccine we turned to Dr. Samuel L. Katz and Dr. Saul Krugman. Dr. Philip A. Brunell brought us up to date on the current status of chicken pox immunization and the use of zoster immune globulin.

Two virologist fathers told us how they isolated important viruses from their children; Dr. Thomas Weller the German measles virus from his son Robert, and Dr. Maurice Hilleman the mumps virus from his daughter Jeryl Lynn. In addition, Dr. Hilleman gave us valuable information on vaccine-making and arranged for us to tour the production facilities of Merck Sharp and Dohme in West Point, Pennsylvania. To Merck, and to Eli Lilly and Co., we are also indebted for technical information and illustrative material.

Dr. W. Charles Cockburn, Mrs. Ruth Cavanaugh, and Mr. L. M. Thapalyal provided us with a wealth of material on the activities of the World Health Organization. Descriptions of mass vaccination procedures came from Dr. Lawrence Altman and from Dr. Pascal Imperato, who was also kind enough to let us use some photographs from his personal files. Several electron micrographs were selected from the laboratory of Dr. Samuel Dales.

Information on cancer and viruses was supplied by the American Cancer Society and by Drs. Thomas Benjamin and Richard Novick, who told us about current concepts of tumor virology and also about the possible uses of viruses in genetic engineering.

And finally, we want to thank Mrs. Kathleen Wasserman for the patience and care with which she typed the final manuscript.

August, 1971   Nancy Rosenberg
                                          Louis Z. Cooper, M.D.

Introduction

On February 27, 1969, the Apollo 9 spacecraft was being readied for an important flight. Its purpose: to test the equipment that was soon to be used in the first lunar landing. Everything went smoothly until the last minute, when all three of the astronauts developed stuffy noses and sore throats. The countdown had to be halted. Putting a man on the moon, it seemed, was a lot easier than curing the common cold.

Most people probably would be even more excited about a cold cure than they were to see the first man walk on the moon. The average American has three or four cold-like illnesses every year. Most of them are mild and cause only a few days of sneezing, coughing, and nasal congestion. Others, like influenza, bronchitis, and pneumonia, are more serious.

If the doctor diagnoses these cases as "a virus," he's probably right. Viruses are tiny microorganisms that are responsible for the great majority of respiratory illnesses. They are also the cause of smallpox, yellow fever, measles, mumps, and polio. And they don't confine their attacks to people. Chickens, mice, tulips, tobacco plants, and bacteria are just a few of the living things that fall victim to the virus.

Viruses are a recent discovery; they were not recognized as agents of disease until the very end of the nineteenth century. Since then, they have been measured, photographed, and analyzed chemically. Scientists have learned to tame some of them, and this has led to the development of protection in the form of vaccines. Probably, you have had the benefit of a number of them already.

But the control of disease is only one part of the virus story. Because of their unique properties, viruses have given scientists their first chance to probe the inner workings of the living cell. The study of viruses is leading to a new understanding of the processes of life itself.

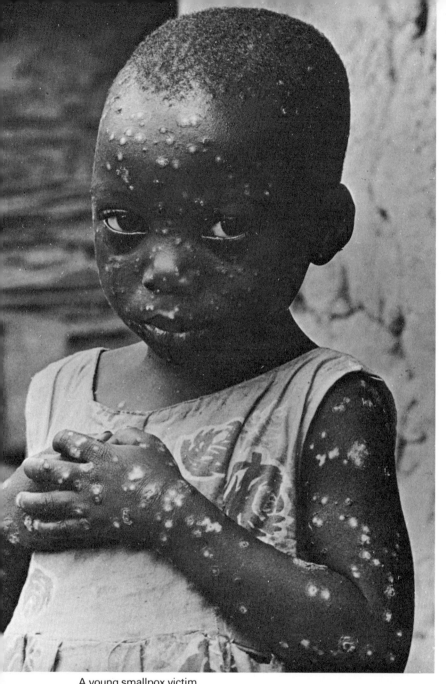

A young smallpox victim.

1

The First Vaccines

When people speak of the good old days, they can't be thinking of medical science. Our ancestors were threatened by diseases that are almost unheard of today. Doctors had no way of preventing these diseases, and there was very little they could do to treat them once they struck.

Smallpox was one of the most terrifying. It killed one person out of every ten and left countless others lame, blind, and deaf. Often, their faces were disfigured with ugly pockmarks. No one knew where smallpox came from or how it spread. Just one thing was certain; it almost never struck the same person twice. Those who had had it were safe for the rest of their lives.

Some cases of smallpox were milder than others. Since nearly everyone had the disease sooner or later, people went out of their way to try to get the mild variety. In fact, they deliberately gave themselves smallpox by a method known as inoculation.

One of the signs of smallpox are blisters, or pustules, that are filled with a clear fluid. Injected under the skin of a healthy person, this fluid can give him smallpox. People were often inoculated with fluid taken from the pustules of patients with mild cases of small-pox. If they were lucky, they had mild cases too.

For the most part, this system worked quite well. Once in a while, though, inoculation produced serious cases. And those who had smallpox by inoculation were just as contagious as those who caught it the natural way.

A much better form of protection was discovered by Edward Jenner, a country doctor in eighteenth century England. Jenner came from the farmlands of Gloucestershire, where there were many cows. Cows are subject to a disease called cowpox, which produces sores on their udders. Sometimes these sores are passed on to the people who milk them.

Jenner had a trait that is shared by all good doctors; he listened carefully to what his patients told him and took their words seriously. One day he was consulted by a young milkmaid. When he suggested that she might be getting smallpox she answered, "I cannot take that disease, for I have had the cowpox." That was a common belief among the country folk; once you had had cowpox, you could never get smallpox. Many doctors scoffed at the idea, but Jenner thought it was worth looking into. He found several people who had had cowpox and tried giving them smallpox by inoculation. Nothing happened.

Then Jenner tried to produce this immunity him-self. When a milkmaid, Sarah Nelmes, came down with cowpox, he took some material from a pustule on her wrist and injected it into the arm of eight-year-old James Phipps. At the site of the injection, James developed redness and a little swelling. A white ring formed, and then a scab. When the scab fell off a few weeks later, nothing was left but a faint round mark.

Six weeks later, James Phipps was inoculated with smallpox. There was no reaction. Over the years, twenty attempts were made to give James Phipps smallpox by inoculation, and all of them failed. In 1798, Jenner published a booklet announcing his discovery. He called it "vaccination," from the Latin word *vacca*, meaning cow. The name stuck, and nowadays all such injections are called vaccinations.

The practice of smallpox vaccination spread quickly, and the disease began to disappear. Jenner was honored far and wide. Today, smallpox is almost unknown in countries where vaccination is practiced.

Although smallpox could now be prevented, its cause was still unknown. Doctors had no idea how cowpox was related to smallpox, or why one disease should prevent another. And they had no way of applying Jenner's discovery to other diseases. Nearly one hundred years had to pass before another vaccine was developed.

The next such discovery was made in France, where the great Louis Pasteur was studying chicken cholera. Germs were well known by Pasteur's time. Pasteur himself had discovered that they were the cause of infectious disease. Scientists were accustomed to examining germs under microscopes and growing them in broths and jellies. Many germs had been identified with the diseases they caused.

Pasteur had succeeded in isolating the germ that causes chicken cholera and getting it to grow in a warm broth. A growth of microorganisms like this one is called a culture. Just a few drops of this culture, injected under the skin, was enough to kill a chicken in a day or two.

In 1879, Pasteur interrupted this work for a summer vacation. When he returned, he injected some chickens with a culture of chicken cholera germs that had been standing around for several weeks. The chickens got sick, but their illness was mild, and before long they recovered completely. Something had gone wrong.

Pasteur cultured a fresh batch of germs and injected a new group of chickens. But he also injected the first group all over again. The new chickens died right on schedule, but the others showed no effects from this second injection. They were immune to chicken cholera! Somehow or other, the first injection had protected them against the second one.

This reminded Pasteur of Jenner and his smallpox vaccination. The culture that had been left standing over the summer was much weaker than the fresh culture. Perhaps the cowpox germ was just a weak relative of the smallpox germ. If this were the case, it should be possible to develop vaccinations for many other diseases.

Pasteur proceeded to do exactly that. He succeeded in vaccinating pigs against swine erysipelas and sheep against anthrax. In each case, he grew the guilty germ, found a way to weaken it, and used the weakened germ as a vaccine.

Then Pasteur turned his attention to rabies, a rare

disease and a horrible one. People get it from the bites of infected animals. These animals carry the rabies germ in their saliva, and if their bite breaks the skin, the germ enters the bloodstream. No symptoms develop for several weeks, but at the end of that time there are convulsions, paralysis, and, inevitably, death.

Pasteur found that he could infect many animals with rabies by injecting them with the saliva of rabid dogs. In one experiment, he worked with a long series of rabbits. Each time a rabbit died of rabies, he injected material from its spinal cord into a healthy rabbit's brain. When he started, the germ took several weeks to make the rabbits sick. But as he worked, the nature of the germ seemed to change, and the rabbits got sick faster and faster. Finally, Pasteur developed a germ that would make a rabbit sick in just six days. He called this process fixation.

These rabbits served the same purpose for Pasteur that the cows had for Jenner. In each case, the germ was changed by its passage through the animal. It could no longer cause disease in people, but it *could* give them protection against its more virulent relative.

Pasteur weakened the rabies germ by storing the infected spinal cord, just as he had stored the culture of chicken cholera germs. The longer he stored the spinal cord, the weaker the rabies germ became. By the end of two weeks, it was too weak to infect a rabbit at all.

Now Pasteur was ready to vaccinate dogs against rabies. It took fourteen injections to do it, starting with the weakest germ and working up, day by day, to the strongest. At the end of that time, the dogs were completely immune.

Pasteur had misgivings about trying this treatment on a human patient, but before long he was forced to. In the summer of 1885, a nine-year-old schoolboy, Joseph Meister, was attacked by a rabid dog. He had many deep bites, and doctors agreed that he would surely get rabies. Pasteur was persuaded to vaccinate him at once.

Joseph Meister received twelve shots of rabies vaccine over an eleven-day period. The great Pasteur was uneasy, but his treatment was a huge success. No symptoms of rabies ever developed in Joseph Meister. When word of this triumph spread, people who had been bitten by rabid animals flocked to Pasteur. Almost 2500 of them were vaccinated during the next fifteen months.

Although Pasteur conquered rabies, he was never able to isolate the germ that caused it. He concluded that the rabies germ was too small to be seen, even under a microscope, and he called it by a Latin name, "*virus*," meaning poison. Pasteur believed that there were many more of these sub-microscopic organisms. Future events would prove that he was right.

2

The Virus Revealed

Scientists often make their discoveries in unexpected places. The first virus, for instance, was recovered from the leaves of a sick tobacco plant.

Tobacco is subject to a disease that mottles its leaves and makes them brittle. The mottling looks something like a mosaic, so the condition is called tobacco mosaic disease. In 1898, a Dutch botanist named Martinus Beijerinck set out to find the germ that causes it.

Beijerinck began by squeezing some juice out of the mottled tobacco leaves. When this juice was rubbed on healthy leaves, they too developed the mottled pattern. The cause of the disease was somewhere in that juice, but when Beijerinck examined a drop of it under his microscope there was not a germ to be seen.

Next, Beijerinck tried to grow the germ. He put some of the juice on a warm plate of agar, a jelly that comes from seaweed. Many germs thrive on it. But the germ that caused tobacco mosaic disease remained as invisible as ever.

Then Beijerinck tried another approach. He poured the infectious juice through a porcelain filter with holes smaller than the smallest germ known. If the liquid that passed through the filter could no longer cause the disease, he would know that he had trapped the germ inside the filter.

This time Beijerinck got the biggest surprise of all. He rubbed the filtered juice on some healthy leaves, and within a few days they too had the mottled pattern. And the juice squeezed from *them* was infectious too. The cause of tobacco mosaic disease, whatever it was, had slipped through the holes in the filter and was still multiplying.

Six years earlier, a Russian botanist, Dimitrii Iwanowski, had performed the same experiment and gotten the same result. He had thought that there must be something wrong with his filters. But Beijerinck reached a different conclusion. Here was an infectious juice that was able to reproduce itself. To do that, it had to be alive. The juice, said Beijerinck, was an entirely new form of life. He called it a *contagium vivum fluidum*, a living, contagious fluid.

Borrowing a term from Pasteur, Beijerinck also spoke of his contagious fluid as a filterable virus. In Pasteur's day, the term virus was used to refer to germs in a general way. But Beijerinck had something very specific in mind. He was talking about a form of life that couldn't be seen under a microscope or grown on a plate of agar. And that is how the term is used today.

Before long, a number of other viruses came to light. More and more diseases seemed to be caused by invisible germs that couldn't be trapped in porcelain filters or grown in laboratory dishes.

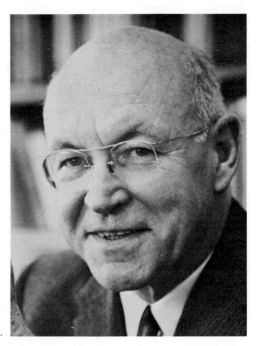

Biochemist Dr. Wendell
M. Stanley, who set out
to isolate the TMV virus.

By 1931 it was clear that Beijerinck had been wrong
about one thing. The "filterable viruses" were not
always filterable. Dr. William J. Elford showed that if
the holes in the filters were small enough, the fluid
that passed through them was no longer infectious. So
viruses were not fluids after all; they were incredibly
small solid particles. As Pasteur had suspected, there
was a whole world of germs beyond the range of the
ordinary microscope.

What were these germs made of? What did they
look like? And how could anything so tiny be alive?
The only way to answer these questions was to separate the virus from the fluid that contained it, and in
1932 a biochemist named Wendell M. Stanley set out
to do just that.

Huge molecules called proteins were receiving a lot of attention at that time. Proteins come in a tremendous variety, and they are found in all living things. Stanley thought that viruses were made of protein too. If they were, he knew that he could isolate them with a long, complicated chemical procedure. The virus would have to be tough to withstand it. It would also have to be safe to work with and easy to detect. All in all, the tobacco mosaic virus, or TMV as it had come to be called, seemed to be the best choice.

Stanley grew a large crop of Turkish tobacco plants. When they were a few inches high, he rubbed their leaves with tobacco mosaic virus. Several weeks later he harvested the sick plants, about a ton of them.

First he froze the plants to rupture their cells. Then he put the frozen plants through a meat grinder, thawed the pulp, and squeezed the juice out of it. From this murky soup, he prepared to extract the virus in pure form.

Stanley filtered, dissolved and precipitated over and over again to separate the various parts of the mixture. To keep track of the virus, he tested each part on the leaves of a healthy tobacco plant. Whatever produced the mottled pattern was kept; the rest was discarded. As he worked, the solution grew paler and paler.

Finally Stanley obtained a shimmering, colorless liquid. Slowly, he added a chemical to it, stirring until the solution grew cloudy. Then added another substance. The liquid developed a satin-like sheen; it had turned into long, slender crystals. There was only a spoonful of them, but they were all that Stanley

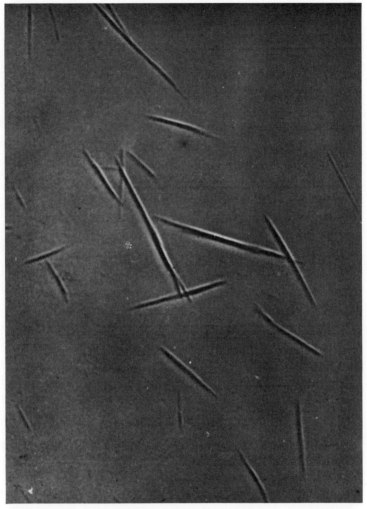

These long, slender crystals of TMV were prepared in Dr. Stanley's laboratory.

wanted. Dissolved in water, they produced the familiar mottled pattern on healthy tobacco leaves. The
needle-like crystals were pure tobacco mosaic virus!

Stanley's discovery created a sensation in the
scientific world. TMV crystals looked very much like
ordinary table salt. Left in a bottle on a laboratory
shelf, there was nothing to distinguish them from
hundreds of perfectly ordinary chemicals. No one
would have thought of calling them alive. They
didn't eat, or move, or show any of the other characteristics of living things. But put in solution and
brushed on a tobacco leaf, they seemed to spring into
life.

Were they dead or alive? What did "alive" really
mean?

These questions touched off a tremendous amount
of investigation. When the answers were in, the virus
turned out to be even more remarkable than anyone
had imagined.

3

The Living Crystal and How to Avoid It

Today's scientists are very much at home in the world of the virus. Once Stanley had shown the way, a number of different viruses were isolated in pure form. With the help of the newly developed electron microscope, it was finally possible to see what they looked like, and a fascinating lot they turned out to be.

The world of the virus is inconceivably small. TMV crystals, for example, are only one hundred-thousandth of an inch long. It would take about 800,000 of them, laid end to end, to go from the top of this page to the bottom. Polio viruses are so small that 25 million of them could fit on the head of a pin. A billion billion would be needed to fill a pong-pong ball. To explore a world this tiny, scientists have had to use giant apparatus. One of their most useful tools has been the electron microscope.

In the electron microscope, a beam of electrons takes the place of visible light. Even though they are solid particles, electrons have a wavelength associated with them, and it is much smaller than that of light.

23

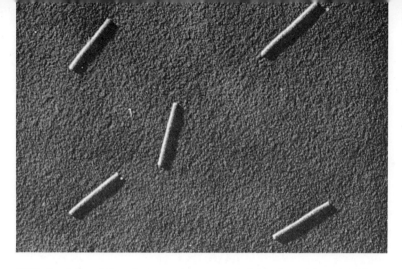

With the help of the electron microscope, individual particles of TMV become visible.

This makes the electron microscope more powerful. It can be used to see particles as small as two hundred-millionths of an inch in diameter.

The polio virus is a tiny sphere. Vaccinia is shaped like a loaf of bread. The T2 bacteriophage looks more like a tadpole. And the adenovirus takes the form of a well-known solid, the icosahedron. It is formed by twenty equilateral triangles put together in space.

Viruses are so small that they are measured in a special unit, the millimicron. A millimicron is one-billionth of a meter, and a meter is a little over 39 inches. The smallest living thing is 150 millimicrons long; the largest known molecule is about 22. Most viruses fall somewhere in between them.

The size of the virus is a clue to its place in the biological scheme of things. Viruses fill the gap between the living and the non-living worlds. One scientist wondered jokingly whether they were "organules or molechisms."

Viruses can grow only in living cells. The cell is the basic unit of all living things, both plant and animal. There are nerve cells and muscle cells, blood cells and bone cells. Each cell contains a tiny drop of a jelly-like substance called protoplasm enclosed in a cell membrane. In plants, the cells have rigid walls as well. All the functions of life take place inside the protoplasm, under the direction of the cell's nucleus, which lies near its center.

Under natural conditions, viruses are very particular about which cells they grow in. The polio virus grows only in the cells of man and his nearest relatives in the monkey family. TMV grows only in certain plants. No wonder Beijerinck couldn't make it grow on plates of agar.

The virus has a dual personality; sometimes it is a harmless crystal, sometimes a killer. In its crystalline state, it is as lifeless as dust. But in an appropriate living cell all this changes. The virus enters the cell and destroys it, sometimes in a matter of minutes. In the process, hundreds of new viruses are produced, all exactly like the first one. For when it comes to reproduction, the virus is a champion.

To understand how a virus reproduces, you must know something about its chemical structure. Stanley's guess that the virus was made of protein was not entirely right. Actually, it is 95% protein and 5% nucleic acid. But this last 5% is extremely important.

There are two kinds of nucleic acid, ribonucleic acid, or RNA, and deoxyribonucleic acid, or DNA. They are called nucleic acids because they were first found in the nuclei of living cells. As more and more

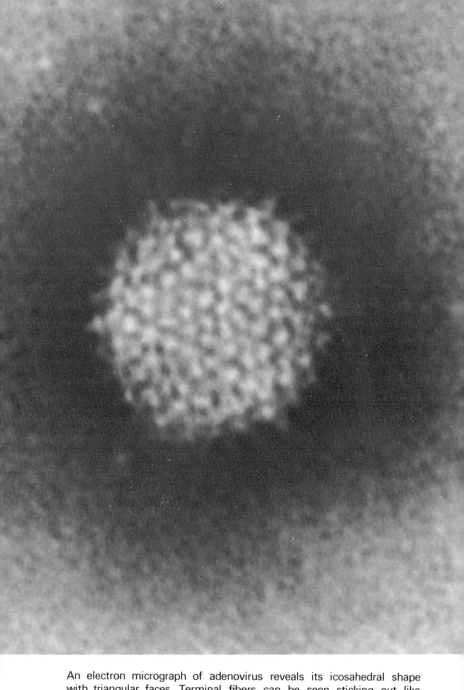

An electron micrograph of adenovirus reveals its icosahedral shape with triangular faces. Terminal fibers can be seen sticking out like antennae from three of the 20 faces. (Magnified 800,000 times).

cells were studied, and all of them were found to contain nucleic acid, it became clear that nucleic acid is a vital component of all living things. In fact, it has turned out to be the key to life itself.

The living cell is a busy place. It carries out a multitude of chemical reactions, all at incredible speeds. Certain substances are broken down; others are manufactured. All of these reactions are controlled by different kinds of DNA in the cell's nucleus. This DNA forms the genes that carry hereditary information from one generation to the next. RNA is the messenger that carries instructions from the DNA to the cell. As the source of this vital information, nucleic acid is really the blueprint of life.

The nucleic acid of the virus is a blueprint too—for making new virus particles. But viral nucleic acid is a blueprint without a cell. It is surrounded only by a protein coat.

When a virus finds a cell it can infect, it attaches itself to the cell wall, makes a hole in it, and squirts its nucleic acid inside. From this moment on, the cell stops taking orders from its own nucleic acid and the viral nucleic acid takes over. Instead of attending to its own needs, the cell devotes its energy to manufacturing and assembling the parts for new virus particles. When the job is finished, the cell bursts open and hundreds of virus particles escape, each ready to infect a cell of its own.

Viruses can produce a host of different symptoms, depending on what kind of cells they infect. There are many possibilities; more than 500 different viruses have been found inside the human body.

Viruses can give you rashes, fevers, swollen glands, and even paralysis. If a virus infects your liver cells, it can turn you yellow with jaundice. When the cells that line your nose fall victim to a virus, you get the sneezing and nasal congestion of a cold. Luckily, the body has a way of defending itself against attacks like these.

When a virus enters the body, it triggers a mechanism known as the immune response. The virus serves as an antigen, a protein with its own special chemical makeup. The body responds to this antigen by manufacturing antibodies, proteins that are especially tailored to fit the antigen in much the same way as a key is tailored to fit a lock. Each antibody attaches itself to a virus and prevents it from entering a cell.

When a virus enters your body for the first time, it infects your cells and makes you ill. But antibodies form rapidly, and as they do you begin to recover. The germs disappear, but not the antibodies; they stay behind to protect you against the particular germ that produced them. That is why people never get diseases like smallpox more than once.

Each organism is different, and each requires its own special antibodies. But there's no limit to the number of these fighting particles you can carry in your bloodstream. Some are the result of bouts you've had with infectious disease. Others are there because a doctor gave you a vaccine that was designed to produce them.

There are two kinds of virus vaccines. Killed virus vaccines are made of viruses that have been killed in such a way that they are no longer able to cause disease. Live virus vaccines are made of viruses that have been weakened, or attenuated, so that, although they are still living, they can no longer make you ill. Your body reacts to these killed or attenuated germs just as it would to their untamed cousins. Antibodies develop, and they stay around to protect you against a disease you've never had. Immunologically speaking, it's a little like having your cake and eating it too.

The first step in making a virus vaccine is catching the virus. Usually it is recovered from someone who has been infected by it. Then a susceptible laboratory animal must be found. Countless animals have been infected with human diseases in the interest of medical science. Monkeys have had measles and polio. Ferrets

An electron micrograph of vaccinia virus which has a shape more like a brick or loaf of bread. (Magnified 170,000 times).

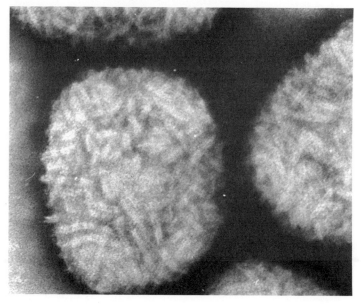

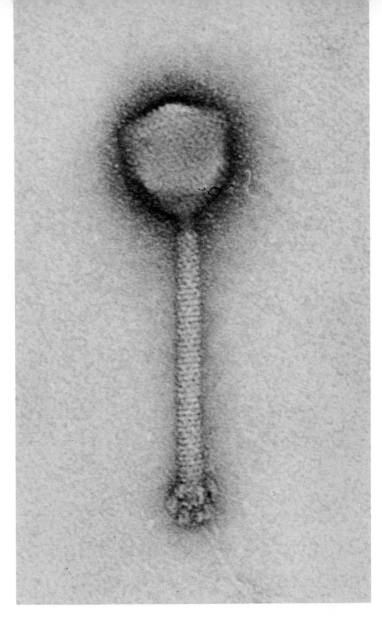

A virus that grows in bacteria is called a bacteriophage. (Magnified about 500,000 times).

have had the flu. By developing the right list of symptoms, these animals serve to identify the virus and to
give an indication of its strength.

Virologists have found that they can attenuate a
virus by adapting it to a new host. If it is accustomed
to growing in human nerve cells, they grow it in cells
from a monkey's kidney. Generation after generation
of viruses are grown in this new host, until the virus is
well adapted to it. As it adapts, it loses some of its
original characteristics, among them the ones that
made it cause disease.

This is what Pasteur accomplished by passing the
rabies germ from rabbit to rabbit. But using animals
as living incubators is expensive and difficult. Today's
virologist is much more likely to grow his virus in a
tissue culture. Tissue cultures are growths of living
cells that are kept alive in laboratory dishes. Viruses
can also be passed through the shells of fertile eggs
and grown in the embryos inside them.

All of these techniques and more are employed in
the making of modern vaccines. Jenner was lucky; in
cowpox he had stumbled on a ready-made smallpox
vaccine. Conquering other diseases has often been a
long and difficult process.

4

Down with the Yellow Jack

For hundreds of years, the ships that plied the Atlantic trade routes sailed under a threat of death. Its symbol was a yellow flag, the notorious "yellow jack" that flew wherever yellow fever raged.

Yellow fever is a disease of the tropics: Africa, South America, and the West Indies. The natives are largely immune to it. They usually get mild cases early in childhood, and having had the disease once, can never get it again. But for visitors from other parts of the world, yellow fever can often be fatal.

A typical case begins with fever, chills, and a headache. Within a few days, the patient develops yellow jaundice and vomits material that is black with blood. Death can follow within a week.

During the Spanish-American War, yellow fever took so many American lives that the United States Army decided to investigate it. A commission headed by Major Walter Reed was sent to Cuba in 1900. They searched for the cause of yellow fever, but were unable to find it.

Walter Reed did a number of experiments with human volunteers in an attempt to discover how yellow fever was spread. He put volunteers in rooms where yellow fever patients had been, but they didn't become ill. They didn't catch yellow fever from the patients' clothing either, or even from the patients themselves. The culprit, it turned out, was an African mosquito, the Aedes *aegypti*. And yellow fever, like rabies and smallpox, was caused by a filterable virus. It was, in fact, the first human disease for which a virus was proven to be the cause.

Before long, the Aedes *aegypti's* role in spreading yellow fever was fully understood. When the mosquito bites, it sucks blood. If its victim is a yellow fever patient, this blood contains yellow fever virus. Once inside the mosquito's body, the virus multiplies for twelve days. From then on, the mosquito infects everyone it bites.

Armed with this knowledge, it was easy to protect people from yellow fever. The Aedes *aegypti* breeds in open containers of water around people's houses. Such containers were outlawed. Those that were absolutely necessary had to be screened or covered with a film of oil. And yellow fever patients were kept under netting for the first three days of their illness. This prevented the mosquitoes from biting them and picking up the virus.

With measures like these, yellow fever soon became a thing of the past. By 1901, it was all but eliminated from Havana. The same precautions, applied in Panama, made possible the building of the Panama Canal. For a while everyone thought the problem was solved. Then it was discovered that yellow fever still raged deep in the jungle.

Man is not the only victim of the yellow fever virus; it infects monkeys too. High in the treetops of the African and South American jungles, mosquitoes carry the virus from monkey to monkey. These jungle mosquitoes are beyond human control. Anyone working near the jungle runs the risk of being infected by them and carrying yellow fever back to civilization.

At this point, the yellow fever story switches from the tropical jungles to the Harvard Medical School in Boston. There, in 1929, Dr. Max Theiler took the first step toward developing a yellow fever vaccine.

At that time, the only laboratory animals that had been found to be susceptible to yellow fever were Rhesus monkeys, and they were very expensive. White mice were cheaper and more plentiful, but no one had been able to infect them with yellow fever. The virus had been injected under their skins and into their abdomens with no observable results. Taking a cue from Pasteur, Theiler tried injecting the yellow fever virus directly into the mice's brains. Within a few days, all of them were dead.

The virus that Theiler injected into the mice had come from the liver of a monkey that had died of yellow fever. The monkey had had a typical case, but the virus affected the mice very differently. They developed none of the usual symptoms of yellow fever. Instead, they died from an inflammation of their brains.

As Theiler passed the virus from one mouse to another, it had a stronger and stronger effect. Finally, the virus became fixed. Injected into the brain of a mouse, this fixed virus was rapidly fatal. But when the same virus was tested on monkeys, it scarcely even made them ill. What it did do was give them immunity to ordinary yellow fever. Theiler had made a yellow fever vaccine for monkeys.

To prove that his fixed virus really was yellow fever,

Theiler developed a "mouse protection test." He made a serum from the blood of people who had recovered from yellow fever. This serum contained yellow fever antibodies. Then he mixed the serum with his virus and injected the mixture into a mouse. The virus alone would have killed the mouse quickly. But if the virus were matched by the antibodies in the serum, they would neutralize it and protect the mouse. And that is exactly what happened.

The mouse protection test could also be used to see whether or not people had antibodies for yellow fever in their blood. A world-wide study was made to find out where yellow fever had been and where it was likely to turn up next.

In the course of his investigations, Theiler himself came down with yellow fever. Fortunately it was a mild case and he recovered quickly, but a number of other workers were not so lucky. Within two years, five of them died from accidental infections. A number of others caught yellow fever but recovered.

In 1934, the French government used Theiler's virus to make the "Dakar scratch vaccine." This was a mixture of smallpox and yellow fever vaccines which was given by scratching it into the skin. Millions received it, and it was extremely effective, but Theiler was far from happy with it. What worried him was the virus' affinity for brain cells, its "neurotropism." He was determined to eliminate it.

A killed virus vaccine for yellow fever was out of the question. Once the yellow fever virus is dead, it no longer stimulates antibody production. The only way to develop a safe vaccine was to get the virus to grow in tissue cultures of non-nervous cells. Theiler worked for several years, passing different strains of virus through flask after flask of minced-up tissue. In one experiment, he used chick embryo with the brain and spinal cord removed. Because it was part of the seventeenth series of experiments he had done, Theiler labeled it 17D.

From time to time, Theiler tested the passaged virus in monkeys to see what effect, if any, the experiment was having. At the beginning, the virus killed any monkey that received it. After about ninety passages, it killed some monkeys, but not all. Soon afterward, it stopped killing monkeys altogether. But it did protect them against the untamed, natural virus.

Theiler had accomplished his goal. He wasn't quite sure how he had done it, and he couldn't make it happen again. But the 17D strain was a safe vaccine, lacking the neurotropism of the Dakar. Dr. Theiler received the Nobel Prize in recognition of the benefit of his discovery to all mankind.

Outbreaks of yellow fever still occur in several parts of the world. More than 200 people died of it in Senegal in 1965, 90% of them children under ten. The following year, there was yellow fever in Argentina, Bolivia and Brazil. Such emergencies are met promptly with both anti-mosquito measures and mass vaccinations. Emergency supplies of vaccine are kept on hand wherever there is danger of yellow fever.

The yellow fever vaccine was just one in a long series of medical achievements. There were many viral diseases to conquer, some of them much closer to home.

5

The Planned Miracle

Not very long ago, summertime meant polio season to worried parents everywhere. Children were kept out of crowds and public places; many were sent away from the city altogether. A killer was on the loose, and no one knew where it would strike next.

There was nothing new about polio. An etching on an old Egyptian tomb shows a young man who had it 4000 years ago. But there *was* something new about polio epidemics. The first had occurred as recently as 1887, when there were 44 cases in Stockholm, Sweden. Seven years later, 132 cases were reported in Vermont. Before long, polio epidemics were an annual event, reaching their peak in late August and early September. One of the worst occurred in 1916, when there were 27,000 polio victims in the United States, 6000 of whom died.

Polio is also called infantile paralysis, because there was a time when it was seen mainly in babies. Before the days of sterilized bottles and modern plumbing, children were exposed to many germs at an early age. Polio was widespread, and nearly all babies had it, usually in a very mild form. Crippling was rare, and most children survived with lifelong immunity.

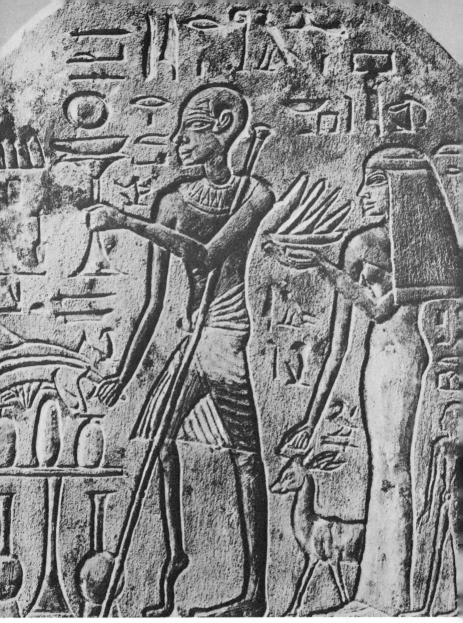

Etching on an Egyptian tomb showing the withered leg of a young polio victim of 4000 years ago.

With the coming of the twentieth century, everything changed. Babies were protected from germs, so they had less chance to develop natural immunity to them. Severe polio became more and more frequent, and the paralysis it caused wasn't "infantile" anymore. Older children and young adults were getting polio too, and for them it was often a serious disease.

Polio is short for poliomyelitis, a name which comes from two Greek words: *polio*, meaning gray, and *myelos*, meaning marrow. It refers to the spinal cord, where polio does its crippling damage.

The brain and the spinal cord together make up the central nervous system. Nerves power muscles, and when nerve cells are destroyed the muscles they control are paralyzed. This paralysis is permanent, because nerve cells cannot regenerate. In time, the useless muscles waste away.

Each part of the nervous system controls a different group of muscles. One portion of the spinal cord sends messages to the arms, another to the legs, and still another to the muscles of the chest and diaphragm which are used for breathing. At the top of the spinal cord, where it enters the brain, is the spinal bulb, a special nerve center that regulates breathing, swallowing, and speech. If enough cells are destroyed in any of these spots, the muscles involved never move again.

Usually polio is not paralytic. Most people who get it don't even feel ill. Others may just have fever, nausea, a sore throat, and a headache. But in some patients, these symptoms are followed by far more serious ones. The headache becomes severe, and is accompanied by vomiting. Then the back and neck grow stiff, and the muscles begin to ache. Soon paralysis sets in. If the patient survives, he may never walk again without braces and crutches. Worse still, he may spend the rest of his life in an iron lung.

One of polio's most famous victims was Franklin Delano Roosevelt, who was stricken in 1921 and paralyzed in both legs. Undaunted, Roosevelt took office twelve years later as the thirty-second President of the United States. He was determined to do something about polio, and in 1938 he helped found the National Foundation for Infantile Paralysis. The Foundation raised millions of dollars to help care for polio patients and to support basic research.

The cause of polio was already known. In 1908, an Austrian physician, Dr. Karl Landsteiner, had injected a monkey with tissue from the spinal cord of a child who had died of polio. Before long, the monkey had fever and paralysis. Dr. Landsteiner found that he could also give monkeys polio by injecting them with fluid taken from the infected spinal cord and passed through a porcelain filter. With this discovery, polio took its place on the growing list of virus diseases. From that day on, there were hopes that a polio vaccine might one day be developed.

For many years, progress in polio research was almost at a standstill. No one could find a reliable way to grow polio virus in the laboratory, and without a large supply of virus there was no hope of making a vaccine. To make matters worse, there was a widespread belief that the polio virus would grow only in nerve cells. If this proved to be the case, the chances of developing a safe vaccine were very poor.

Dr. Karl Landsteiner transmitted polio to monkeys in 1908.

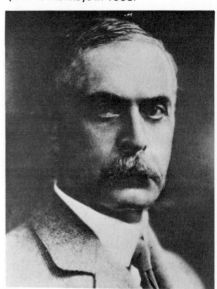

Former President Franklin D. Roosevelt, a famous polio victim, at Warm Springs, Ga. After infection by polio, his legs were less muscular than his arms.

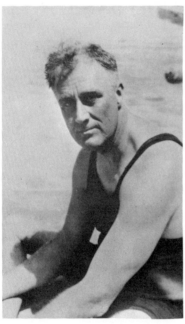

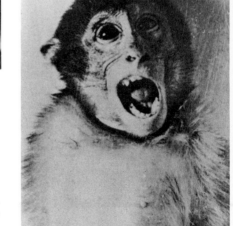

This monkey's face was paralyzed by polio in a laboratory experiment.

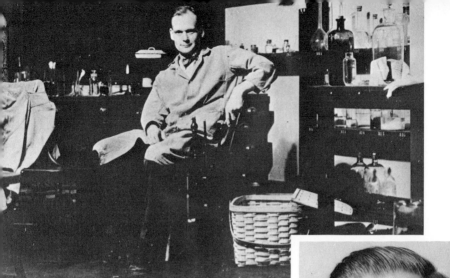

Dr. John F. Enders in his laboratory at Harvard Medical School during the early 1930's.

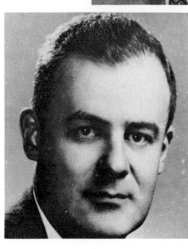

Dr. Thomas H. Weller.

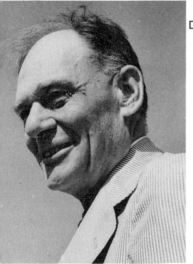

Drs. Enders, Weller and Robbins made a discovery that won them the Nobel Prize. They found that they could grow polio virus in a test tube on non-nervous tissue.

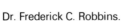

Dr. Frederick C. Robbins.

The real beginning of the end of the polio problem came in 1927, when a young graduate student in the English Department at Harvard decided that microbiology was much more interesting than ancient Germanic languages. John F. Enders was nearly thirty when he joined the Harvard freshmen for courses in elementary chemistry. A few years later, he had a laboratory of his own in the Department of Bacteriology and Immunology at Harvard Medical School.

John Enders is still at Harvard, but today he is a Nobel laureate. His office is decorated with pictures of Edward Jenner, Robert Koch, and Louis Pasteur, men whose work he carried forward with major contributions of his own. For it was Dr. Enders and his team who first found a reliable way to grow viruses, simply and easily, in a test tube.

At the time of their great success with polio in 1948, Dr. Enders and his two young associates, Dr. Thomas H. Weller and Dr. Frederick C. Robbins, were really concentrating on mumps and chicken pox. Under a grant from the National Foundation, they were trying to grow these viruses in tiny bits of tissue suspended in a nutrient medium. In one experiment, Tom Weller was growing chicken pox virus in tissue from a human embryo.

This technique for growing viruses had been originated in 1928 by a husband and wife team, Hugh and Mary Maitland. Back in those days, the only way to keep the cultures free of bacteria was to move them to clean flasks every three or four days. But by 1948, the same "wonder drugs" that were curing people of bacterial infections were helping to prevent bacterial growths in tissue cultures. Dr. Weller chose two of them, penicillin and streptomycin, and added them to the cultures in his flasks.

When Dr. Weller had used up his chicken pox virus, he found that he had a few flasks left over. It seemed a shame to waste them, especially since there was a tube of polio virus in the laboratory freezer. By this time there was reason to believe that in the body the polio virus might grow in cells that were not part of the nervous system. Perhaps it would grow in tissue cultures of non-nervous cells as well. So Weller added some polio virus to the extra flasks and waited to see what would happen. He did not have to wait long.

In just a few weeks, it was clear that the polio virus was multiplying in the embryonic tissue. And soon the Enders team was able to show that it would multiply in a number of other types of tissue as well. Far from growing only in nerve cells, polio virus seemed to grow almost anywhere, in skin, in muscle, and in human intestine.

There was just one problem with the suspended tissue cultures. The only way to be sure that the virus was really growing in them was to draw off the fluid, inject it into monkeys, and see if they developed paralysis. Dr. Enders realized that to have a really practical method for growing the virus there would have to be some way of *seeing* the effect that the virus had on the cells. So he used another technique in which the cells grew in thin sheets on the glass walls of the culture tube and could easily be seen under an ordinary microscope. A day or two after polio virus was added to these cultures, the cells first changed their shape and then fell apart because they had been infected and killed by the virus.

It really was quite an achievement. The Enders team had freed virologists of their dependence on mice, monkeys, and other laboratory animals. At the same time, they had opened the way for the long dreamed of polio vaccine.

At about this same time, another important discovery was announced by a group of researchers at Johns Hopkins University in Baltimore. They had tested nineteen different strains of polio virus and found that all of them fell into one of three groups, each with its own special antibodies. During the next three years, the National Foundation's Committee on Typing painstakingly tested one hundred strains, and confirmed these results. There were just three types of polio virus; a vaccine containing all of them would provide complete protection.

Now the final push was on. The National Foundation decided to develop a killed virus vaccine, and the man they called upon to do it for them was Dr. Jonas E. Salk. Dr. Salk had already helped to develop a killed virus vaccine for influenza. He had had experience with the polio virus too, as a member of the Committee on Typing.

There were many decisions to be made. The polio virus could now be grown in a number of different kinds of cells. Which would be the best? Dr. Salk decided to use monkey kidney cells, and in 1951, at the University of Pittsburgh, he grew three strains of polio virus in them, one for each of the major types.

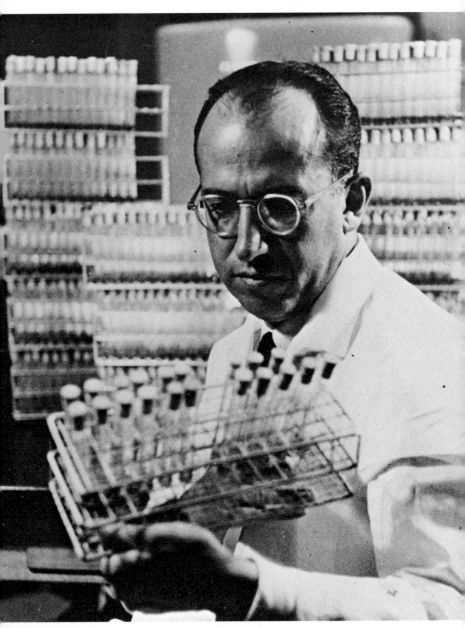

Dr. Jonas E. Salk working to develop the polio vaccine.

The next step was to find the best way to kill the virus. Dr. Salk planned to do this by exposing the infected tissue cultures to formaldehyde. But how much formaldehyde should be used, and how long should the exposure be? These were crucial questions. Too much formaldehyde for too long, and the virus might be too weak to stimulate antibody production. Too little for too short a time, and the vaccine could be dangerous. In the end, Dr. Salk arrived at just the right "recipe." It took him three years of hard work to do it.

Just to be on the safe side, Dr. Salk tried his vaccine out first on some children who had been crippled by polio. They already had polio antibodies, of course, but after receiving the vaccine they had even more. During the next two years, 12,000 people received the Salk vaccine, among them Dr. Salk's three young sons, Peter, Darrell, and Jonathan.

In 1954, Dr. Thomas Francis directed a huge field trial in which two million children took part. Some received the Salk vaccine; others got a harmless salt solution that looked just like it. No one knew which was which until the trial was over. In April, 1955, when the results were in, it was clear that the Salk vaccine was a great success. Statistics showed that it had prevented paralytic polio 80 to 90% of the time. For Dr. Francis, who had trained Dr. Salk fifteen years before, the outcome was especially satisfying. Basil O'Connor, the president of the National Foundation, called the vaccine a "planned miracle."

Even though the Salk vaccine was both safe and effective, many doctors thought a live vaccine would

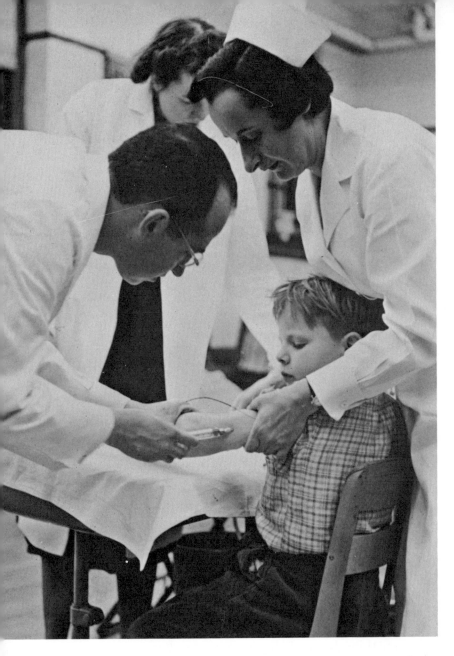

Dr. Salk giving a boy a polio vaccine shot during one of the early trials.

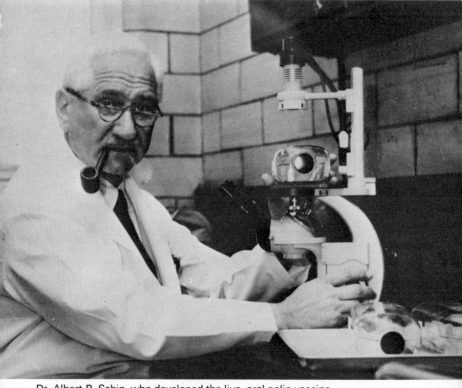

Dr. Albert B. Sabin, who developed the live, oral polio vaccine.

be even better. By the late 1950's, Dr. Albert B. Sabin, of the University of Cincinnati, had developed one. Dr. Sabin's vaccine has many advantages. The Salk vaccine requires three injections; the Sabin vaccine is given orally on a sugar cube or in a glass of water. Since the vaccine virus is alive, it multiplies inside the body, just as the natural polio virus would. Immunity develops quickly, and it probably lasts for life. Because it is alive, the vaccine virus spreads from one person to another, and protection from polio

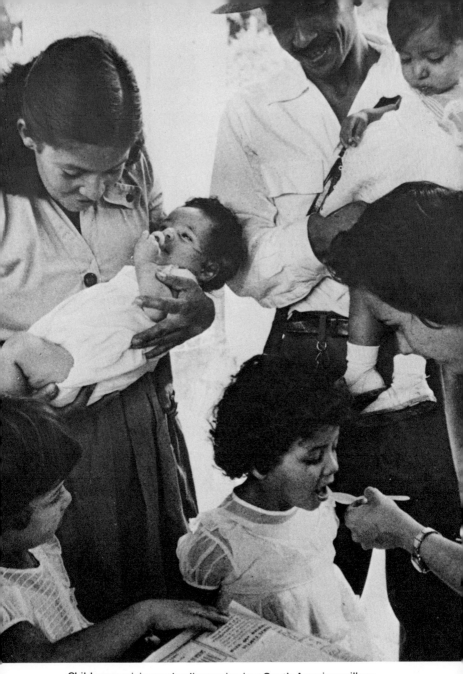
Children receiving oral polio vaccine in a South American village.

spreads with it. These features make the oral vaccine especially useful in preventing epidemics.

Today polio is a vanishing disease. Before the days of the Salk and Sabin vaccines, the United States had as many as 30,000 cases of polio a year, sometimes even more. By 1967 the figure was down to just 40. Many people must share the credit for this achievement, but outstanding among them are John Enders and his co-workers at Harvard. Everything depended on their discovery of a practical method for growing polio virus in non-nervous tissue.

Dr. Enders' contribution to medical science didn't end with his solution of the polio problem. Within ten years, a second breakthrough in Dr. Enders' laboratory would lead to the conquest of another important viral disease.

6

Measles: A Vicious Virus

Near the village of Zoom, on the Volta-Mali border in West Africa, an American doctor pitched his tent and settled down to a supper of wild guinea. Night fell, and presently, through the darkness, the village elders brought him five small children. By the light of a kerosene lamp, he inoculated the children with measles vaccine. Not a tear was shed. Suddenly the doctor heard footsteps all around him. The entire village had been watching, and everyone wanted a measles shot.

This was in March, 1963, and the doctor was Harry Meyer of the United States Public Health Service. He had brought the measles vaccine to West Africa because that was where people needed it most. In Africa, measles usually strikes babies under two, and it is much more of a problem in infants this age than it is in older children. Complications are likely to develop and are more serious when they do. There are parts of Africa and South America where measles is responsible for more than half the deaths among infants. No wonder the people of Zoom were so anxious to be protected against it.

Even in the United States, measles is more serious than many people realize. Before a measles vaccine was available, more than nine out of ten children caught measles, half of them before they were five. Measles starts with a high fever, a runny nose, a cough, and a sore throat. After five days, a blotchy red rash develops. Usually the disease runs its course in another week, but sometimes there are complications. One measles patient in every six develops pneumonia or a serious ear infection. One in every thousand gets measles encephalitis, an inflammation of the brain that can cause paralysis, mental retardation, and even death. Far from being a "harmless childhood disease," measles kills more children than any other acute infectious illness.

Epidemics of measles occur whenever there is a large group of susceptible children. This is likely to be every two or three years in the United States, and even more often in countries where the birth rate is higher. When those who carry the virus have frequent encounters with those who can catch it from them, the disease spreads rapidly. Each case of measles confers lifelong immunity, so as more and more children catch it, less and less are susceptible, and the epidemic begins to taper off. But measles never dies out completely. Susceptible people are always in danger of getting it.

Measles was first described by Rhazes, an Arabian physician, in A.D. 900. Throughout history, many different remedies have been prescribed for it. Adder's tongue, serpent's tongue, bistort, and snakeweed were recommended in seventeenth century England. Today we know that measles, like all virus diseases, cannot be treated effectively once it strikes. Prevention is the only safeguard against it.

The first person who tried to prevent measles by inoculation was Francis Home, an eighteenth century Scottish physician. In Home's time, measles was a serious illness in Scotland, just as it is in parts of Africa today. It was his idea to use inoculation to make "the disease more mild and safe in the same way as . . . . . (we) mitigate the smallpox." But there was a problem. As Home put it, there was "no matter to be had from the measles." Unlike smallpox, measles produced no sores from which material suitable for inoculation could be taken.

Finally Home decided to use blood taken from measles patients at the height of their illness, just after the rash had broken out. He inoculated twelve children. Of the twelve, ten developed fever and coughing six or seven days after inoculation, and a rash several days after that.

Others tried to reproduce Home's results with varying degrees of success, but inoculation against measles was never widely practiced. In the light of recent discoveries, though, it seems likely that Home did succeed in giving measles by inoculation.

Before there was a vaccine for measles, a technique something like Home's was used to lessen its severity. Gamma globulin, the fraction of the blood that contains the antibodies, was sometimes given to susceptible children who had been exposed to measles. Nearly everyone has measles sooner or later, so most people have measles antibodies in their blood. A child who got gamma globulin usually had a mild case of measles, free of complications.

Gamma globulin was all right as far as it went, but the protection it provided was only temporary. To solve the measles problem once and for all, an effective vaccine was needed. The discovery that led to one was made in 1954 in the laboratory of Dr. John Enders, the man with a green thumb for virus-growing.

Dr. Enders had been working with the measles virus on and off for twenty-five years because, as he says, "it was a challenge." Proof that measles is a virus disease had come in 1911 when Dr. Joseph Goldberger filtered blood from a measles patient and used it to pass the disease on to a monkey. In 1938, Dr. Harry Plotz succeeded in cultivating the virus in tissue cultures of chick embryo cells, but his work could not be reproduced, and the presence of the virus was difficult to detect.

At first, Dr. Enders' luck was no better. Then, in 1954, after his triumph with the polio virus, he decided to have another go at measles. In January of that year, measles broke out at the Fay School in nearby Southboro. A number of the boys there caught it, but one of them, David Edmonston, was destined to go down in medical history. When Dr. Thomas Peebles, an associate of Dr. Enders, arrived to examine David, he found him with a full-blown case of measles. Dr. Peebles took some of David's blood and throat washings and hurried back to his laboratory. There he injected the specimens into a culture of human kidney tissue and waited for something to happen.

Within a few days, something did. The appearance of the kidney cells began to change. Some of them became much bigger than the others. These "giant cells" had been observed before in children with measles. Here in the tissue culture, their presence was a sign that the virus was multiplying in the cells and destroying them.

The Edmonston strain, as it came to be called, was passed from one tissue culture to another, with the same effect each time. The virus continued to multiply, and the giant cells were always there to prove it. The growth of the virus could be stopped too, with immune serum from the blood of patients who were recovering from measles. This was proof positive; a virus that is neutralized by measles antibodies has to be measles virus. And sure enough, monkeys injected with the Edmonston strain developed typical cases of measles.

Now came the long, hard job of attenuating the virus. Dr. Enders and his team passed it through twenty-four cultures of human kidney tissue. Then they switched it to tissue cultures derived from human amnion, one of the membranes that contains the unborn child, and passed it through twenty-eight cultures of that. From human amnion it went through six passages in chick amnion tissue cultures and fourteen in chick embryo cells.

Finally, more than three years after David Edmonston's case of measles, the Enders team had the virus where they wanted it. Injected in a susceptible monkey, it now produced no outward signs of measles. But it did stimulate the monkey to develop measles antibodies, fully capable of neutralizing unattenuated measles virus.

The investigators had learned all they could from monkeys; now it was time to test the new vaccine on people. Dr. Enders is not a physician, but among his co-workers was an outstanding young pediatrician, Dr. Samuel L. Katz. Dr. Katz was responsible for the next important step, testing the vaccine in children.

The first trial, carried out in 1960 in a Massachusetts school, showed that children reacted to the measles vaccine very differently than monkeys did. Many developed fever; some had a rash. But none were as sick as they would have been with real measles. Their symptoms passed quickly, and in no case were there any complications.

At another school, the vaccine was put to what Dr. Enders has called "the final test," exposure to real measles. Of forty measles-susceptible children there, twenty were given the vaccine and twenty went without it. When a measles epidemic broke out a few months later, 90% of the unvaccinated children caught measles, but those who had received the vaccine were fully protected. This was the first good evidence that one shot of measles vaccine gave solid protection.

Other trials were carried out in countries where measles was a serious problem; Upper Volta, Nigeria, and Israel. Later, a more attenuated vaccine was developed, one that caused less fever and less rash. And in March, 1963, nine years after the measles virus first began to multiply in Dr. Enders' laboratory, a safe, effective measles vaccine was licensed in the United States. The year before, measles had taken the lives of 408 American children; now it need never claim another victim. A single shot provided lifelong protection.

The measles vaccine has had a dramatic effect on the measles problem in the United States. Before the days of the vaccine, four million American children got measles every year. Five years after the vaccine was licensed, only 25,000 cases were reported.

There was just one setback in the victory over measles. While work was underway on the live measles vaccine, a killed measles vaccine was also being developed. Tests showed that this killed vaccine was an effective antibody producer, and it was licensed at the same time that the live one was. Several million children received it.

Two years later, a strange thing happened. Measles broke out, and some of the children who had been given the killed vaccine were exposed to it. They became very ill, with a form of measles that had never been seen before. Their fever was unusually high, and they had a severe rash that didn't look like the rash of regular measles. Their hands and feet were swollen, and they had fluid in their lungs. Instead of protecting them, the killed vaccine had made them sicker than they would have been without any vaccination at all.

Until this happened, many doctors had considered killed vaccines safer than live ones. But what is true for one vaccine is not necessarily true for another. Each virus presents problems and challenges all its own.

7

Chicken Pox and Mumps: Two Milder Ones

Chicken pox is one of the few common diseases of childhood for which there is still no vaccine. There may well never be one. The chicken pox virus plays a peculiar form of hide and seek that many doctors believe makes it a poor candidate for a vaccine.

The chicken pox virus is responsible for two entirely different diseases. In children, it causes the familiar chicken pox, a mild illness with few complications. In adults it causes zoster, a blistering rash on areas of skin that are served by the same nerve roots.

Zoster is an aftermath of chicken pox. When a child recovers from chicken pox, the virus can go into hiding, only to turn up years later in the form of zoster. That is why a chicken pox vaccine is such a poor idea; vaccinating children against chicken pox might mean giving them a case of zoster sometime in the future. Since chicken pox is so mild, it just isn't worth the risk.

There's one group of children who do need protection against chicken pox. These are children with rheumatic fever, leukemia, or any illness that has to be treated with cortisone. In these children, chicken pox doesn't taper off in the usual way. Instead, it continues to spread. Sometimes it can be fatal.

To protect these children, doctors prepare a serum from the blood of people who are recovering from chicken pox or zoster. Called zoster immune globulin, or ZIG, this serum has a high concentration of chicken pox antibodies. When susceptible children are exposed to chicken pox, ZIG can keep them from getting it.

Chicken pox may be here to stay, but mumps is very much on the run. An effective mumps vaccine has been available since 1968.

The mumps vaccine dates from April, 1963, when a Pennsylvania schoolgirl named Jeryl Lynn Hilleman woke up one night with a headache and a high fever. With the light on, it was easy to see why. There were large, tender swellings on either side of Jeryl Lynn's face. She had a typical case of mumps.

Jeryl Lynn's father, Dr. Maurice Hilleman, is one of the world's outstanding virologists. The next morning, when he went to his job as Director of Virus and Cell Biology Research at the Merck Institute for Therapeutic Research in West Point, Pennsylvania, he took swabbings from Jeryl Lynn's throat with him. Perhaps they could supply the virus for a much-needed mumps vaccine.

Mumps has been around for a long, long time. Hippocrates, the famous Greek physician, described a mumps epidemic that struck an island off the coast of Thrace about 2500 years ago. "Swellings

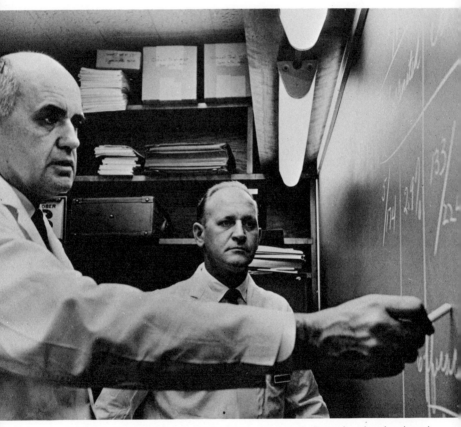

Dr. Maurice R. Hilleman (left) and Dr. Eugene B. Buynak, who developed the live mumps virus vaccine, known as the Jeryl Lynn strain, named for Dr. Hilleman's daughter.

appeared about both ears," he wrote, "in many on either side, and in the greatest number on both sides . . . ." Hippocrates noticed many of the same things abou mumps that we do; it is highly contagious, frequently mild, and sometimes followed by complications.

Mumps starts suddenly with fever, weakness, headache, earache, and difficulty in chewing and swallowing. Then come the swellings of the parotids, a pair of salivary glands that lie below the ears and just in front of them. These swellings last from seven to ten days.

If the patient is lucky, his mumps disappears in about two weeks, never to return again. If he isn't, he can have a wide variety of complications. Mumps can infect the brain, the ears, the eyes, the heart, the joints, the pancreas, and the kidneys. Severe and permanent deafness is one, fortunately rare, complication of mumps. Far more frequent is orchitis, an infection of the male sex glands. Sometimes men and adolescent boys who get orchitis are unable to father children later.

That the cause of all these problems was a virus was established in 1934. By 1943 the mumps virus had been isolated, and two years later it was cultivated in the laboratory. A killed mumps virus vaccine was developed and later, in 1946, Dr. John Enders succeeded in attenuating the mumps virus by passing it through tissue cultures of chick embryo cells. This led to the development of a live mumps virus vaccine as well.

There was just one problem with these vaccines; the immunity they produced didn't last very long. In Russia, a live mumps vaccine has been in use since 1954, and over one million children have received it. But antibody levels drop rapidly, and booster shots are needed. With mumps, this is a serious disadvantage. Because of the threat it poses to men and boys, permanent immunity is especially important.

Dr. Hilleman was able to overcome this difficulty with the virus he took from his daughter Jeryl Lynn. This particular strain, he found, could be attenuated with just a few passages through embryonic egg tissue. Although too weak to cause a real case of mumps, it was strong enough to produce solid immunity which appeared to be long lasting.

The Jeryl Lynn strain was tested on Philadelphia schoolchildren during the fall, winter and spring of 1965-66. Of the 402 who received it, 98% developed mumps antibodies. None had had antibodies before being vaccinated.

Sometime later, a mumps epidemic hit Philadelphia. This put the vaccine to a real test, and it passed with flying colors. Almost none of the vaccinated children got mumps, but half the children in an unvaccinated group came down with it. And the antibody levels in the vaccinated children were almost as high two years later as they had been a month after vaccination. The vaccine seemed to provide the same immunity as a natural case of mumps would.

When the Jeryl Lynn strain live, attenuated mumps virus vaccine was finally licensed in January, 1968,

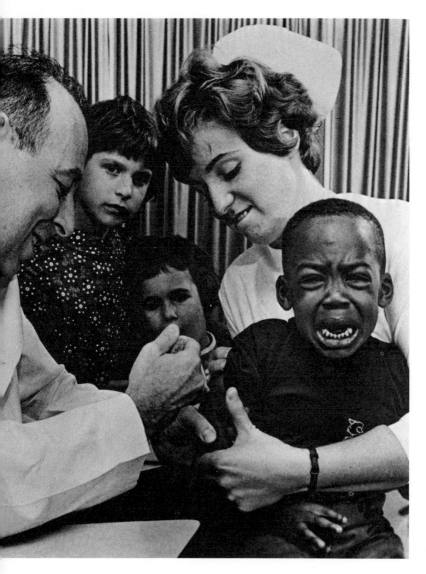

A Philadelphia boy receiving the live mumps virus vaccine.

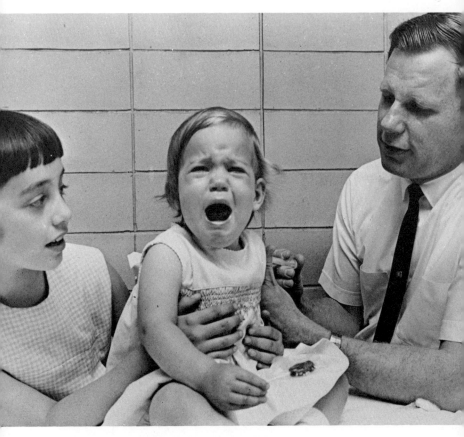

Kirsten Jeanne Hilleman receiving mumps vaccine while being held by her sister, Jeryl Lynn. Their father made the vaccine from a virus he isolated when Jeryl Lynn had the mumps.

one of the first to receive it was Kirsten Jeanne Hilleman, Jeryl Lynn's little sister. For the first time in medical history, one sister was able to protect another from an illness by having it herself.

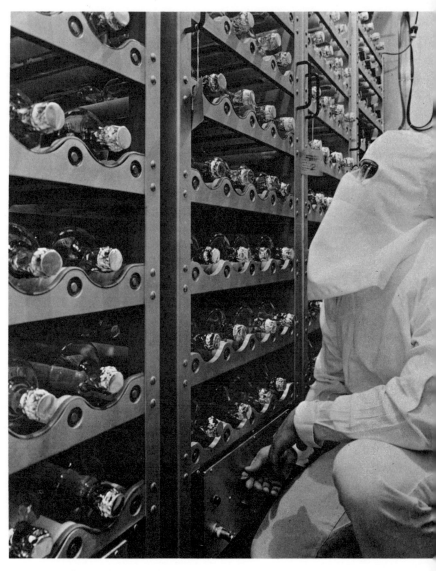

Motorized racks rotate the bottles slowly so that the sheets of cells growing inside them are continually bathed in a nutrient fluid.

8

Vaccine-Making

Row upon row of bottles, lying on their sides, turn slowly on motorized racks. The racks stretch from ceiling to floor and run the full length of a good-sized room. They are tended by a man in a white suit, with a hood that covers most of his face. Only his eyes can be seen, peering at the bottles through heavy goggles. A scene from some brave new world? No, just a production unit in one of the many pharmaceutical companies that manufacture virus vaccines.

Each of these bottles is a breeding place for viruses. Along its inside wall is a layer of the living cells viruses need to grow in. The cells are nourished by a fluid that washes over them as the bottles turn. While the cells grow on the sides of the bottles, the viruses grow inside the cells.

The production unit is just one of many departments involved in the manufacture of vaccines. Vaccine-making is a long, complicated process. It can involve as many as forty different operations and take up to six months to complete. More than two-thirds of this time is spent on rigid quality controls that are built into each step of the manufacturing

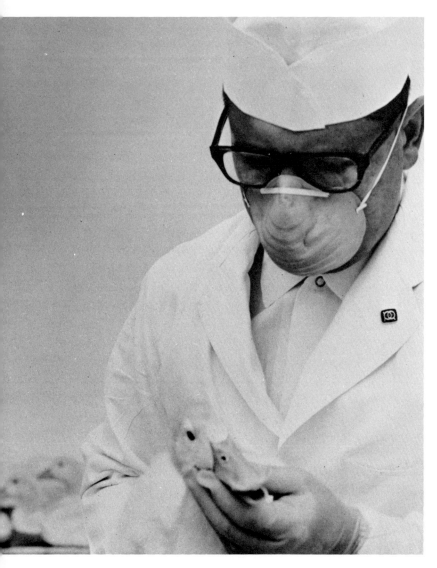

Cell tissue from the embryos of Pekin ducks is used for virus vaccine cultivation. The ducks' private swimming pool is in the background.

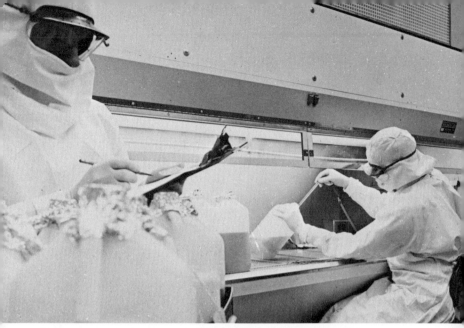

Sanitary garments are worn by workers, and air flow is carefully controlled and filtered whenever vaccine bottles are opened.

process. Every possible precaution is taken to insure that the vaccine will be pure, safe, and effective.

Plants that manufacture vaccines are as germ-free as a modern operating room. Like doctors and nurses, the workers in these plants wear masks, gowns, and gloves. They handle the vaccines under special hoods that control the air flow to prevent contamination. Giant ovens sterilize every instrument and container they use.

The vaccine-making process begins with the cells that the virus will grow in. These too must be as germ-free as it is possible to make them. To be sure that they are, pharmaceutical companies must often breed animals in very special ways.

At the Merck Sharp & Dohme Laboratories in

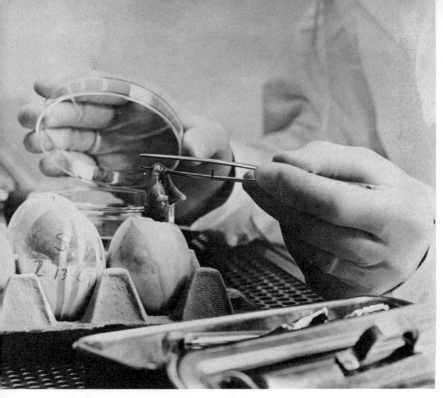

Embryos are removed from the Pekin duck eggs as a first step in preparing tissue culture cells.

West Point, Pennsylvania, a flock of "lucky ducks" enjoy their own private swimming pool. Their quarters, white-walled and sterile, are designed to keep them free of all disease. The air is triple-filtered, and the sawdust on the floor is vacuumed every day. No one is allowed to visit the ducks, and the workers who care for them wear surgical garb.

The purpose of all this special treatment is to produce duck eggs that are absolutely germ-free. The virus that causes German measles grows especially well in the cells of duck embryos. And since ducks are

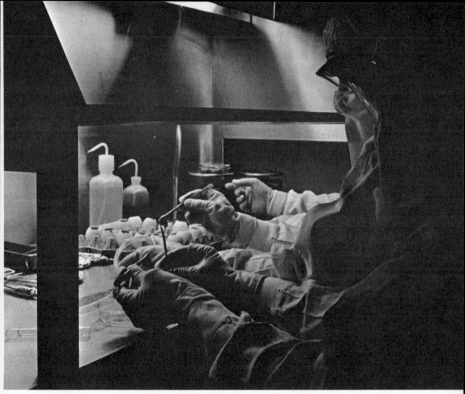

Under a sterile hood the embryos are minced, washed and trypsinized to break them down into individual cells. Then the cells are grown in a nutrient fluid.

unusually healthy animals, duck cell cultures are not likely to be contaminated with unwanted viruses or other organisms. This makes them especially safe for vaccine-making.

The eggs laid by the "lucky ducks" are incubated for fourteen days. Then the embryonic tissue is removed, minced and "trypsinized" to break it down into individual cells. Some of these cells are inoculated into monkeys to check for contamination. The rest are put into bottles with a nutrient fluid and placed on the motorized racks.

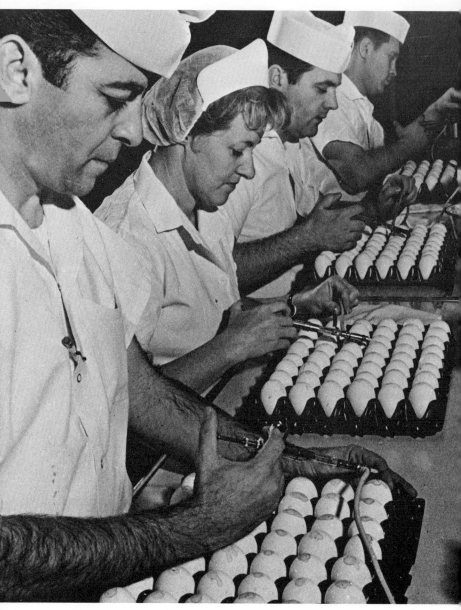
Technicians use special hypodermic syringes to inoculate each hen's egg with seed virus.

For eight days the cells grow on the sides of the bottles. Then, to all but a few of them, a seed virus is added. The unseeded cultures are used as controls; they go through the manufacturing process just as though they had been seeded like the rest. Then they are tested for impurities as a further check on the duck cell cultures.

As the virus grows inside the cells, it is discharged into the nutrient fluid. From time to time this fluid is harvested and replaced with a fresh supply. The fluid containing the virus is pooled and stored in enormous freezers at very low temperatures while samples of it are tested. Only when these tests have been completed is it thawed, subdivided into individual vials, and freeze-dried.

Some vaccines are grown in hens' eggs. Like the ducks, the hens that lay these eggs are kept in spotless surroundings. Each egg's history is recorded on a computerized card so that if any problem should occur it can be traced to a particular hen or rooster.

After eleven days of incubation, the eggs are injected with the virus. Then they are incubated for two days more. During this time, the virus multiplies in the embryonic tissue inside the egg and collects in the fluid around it. The eggs are candled to make sure their embryos are still alive. Eggs with dead embryos are discarded; the others are refrigerated at near-freezing temperatures to stop the growth of the virus. This done, the fluid is harvested, treated with a chemical to concentrate the virus, and whirled around in a centrifuge to separate the virus from the fluid.

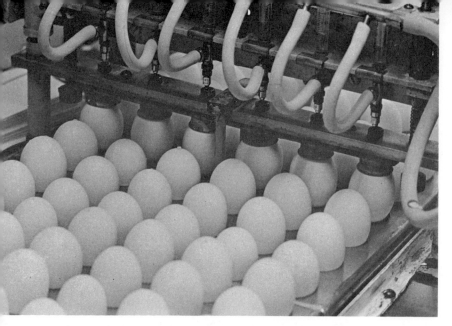

Automatic devices can also be used to inoculate the eggs.

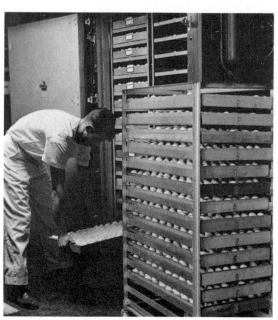

After inoculation, the eggs are incubated for another forty-eight hours to allow the virus to grow inside them.

Then the eggs are candled to make sure the embryos are still alive.

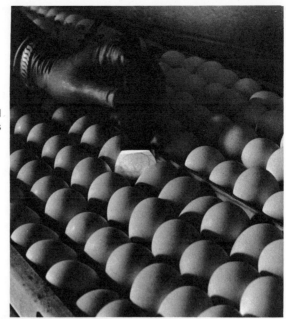

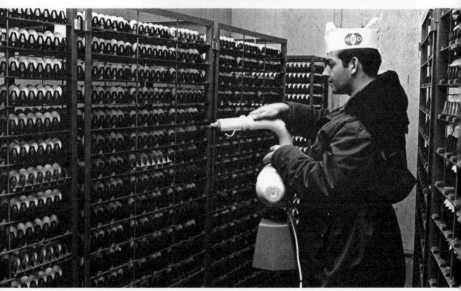

After candling, the eggs are refrigerated in a cold room to stop the growth of the virus. This man is sterilizing the eggs with a disinfectant spray.

Because they are made from living organisms, vaccines are classified as biologics. As such, they are subject to strict government control. A special branch of the Public Health Service, the Division of Biologics Standards, is charged with the responsibility of establishing and maintaining the standards of quality and safety that have been set for biological products. No vaccine can be licensed for distribution to the public until these standards have been met.

When an investigator has developed a virus strain that he thinks might make a good vaccine, he applies to the Division of Biologics Standards for permission to use it on people on an experimental basis. This application is called an IND, an Investigational New Drug application. Included in the IND is a wealth of data; the source of the vaccine, the method for making it, and a description of its physical and chemical properties.

The new vaccine must be tested extensively on laboratory animals to make sure that it has no adverse effects. Its safety established, the potency of the vaccine must be determined. Do animals respond to it by developing antibodies? And do these antibodies afford protection against the unattenuated virus? Only when all these questions have been answered can the vaccine be tried on people.

Volunteers who are inoculated with an experimental vaccine must understand the risk involved and sign a written consent. Vaccines to be used in children must be tested in children; in this case the consent is signed by the parent.

The first trials, carried out on groups of ten or

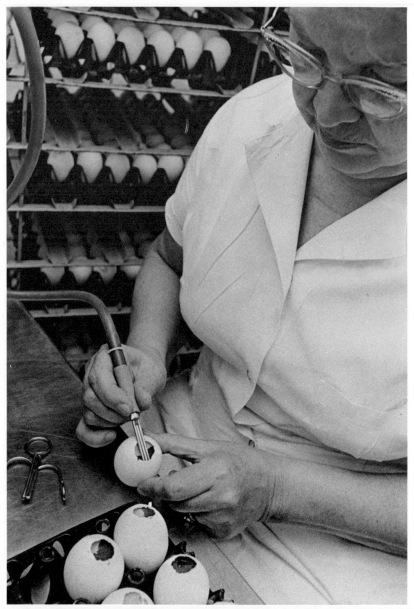

The tops of the eggs are sheared off so that the fluid containing the virus can be drawn out and collected in bottles.

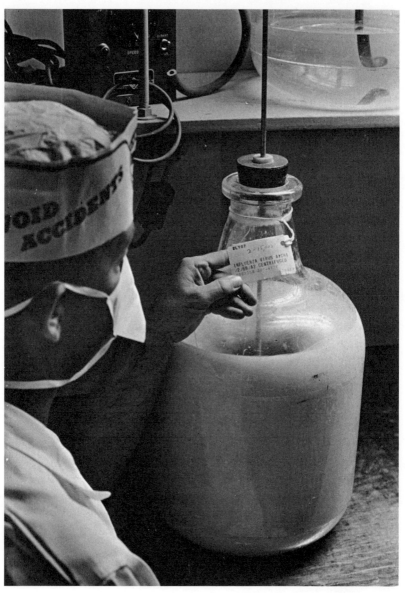

The egg fluid is treated to concentrate the billions of virus
particles inside it.

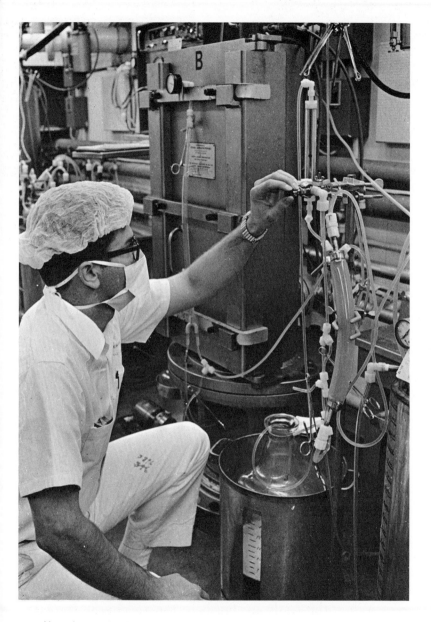
Here the vaccine is being purified in a high speed centrifuge.

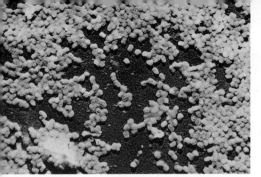

This electron micrograph shows influenza virus vaccine which has been purified in the ultracentrifuge.

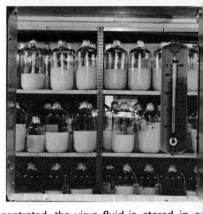

After being concentrated, the virus fluid is stored in c[ ] vaults to await the results of testing for safety and poten[ ] If it passes the tests, it is put in vials and stored until [ ] proval to distribute it has been received from the Divis[ ] of Biologics Standards.

less, can be nerve-racking experiences. In the words of one seasoned investigator, "It's always a difficult thing to try a vaccine on children for the first time. You've experimented with it again and again, and you're sure that it's safe, but you're the one who has to put the needle in that arm, and you have many sleepless nights after you do it. You know that even if they have a mild reaction the real disease would make them sicker, but even so you can't help worrying."

If the first trials are successful, they are expanded to include hundreds of people, then thousands. Before a vaccine can be licensed, it must prove to be safe and potent for a specified number of susceptible individuals. This number varies with the severity of the illness involved. For a mild disease like mumps, it is 5000; for polio, one million inoculations are required.

When the trials are finished, the vaccine is turned over to commercial pharmaceutical companies.

Developing a vaccine in the laboratory is one thing; finding ways to mass-produce it safely and efficiently is quite another. Sometimes years are required to develop the production methods and controls that are needed before a vaccine can be made available to the public.

Even after a vaccine has been licensed, the government keeps a watchful eye on it. Every year, special members of the DBS staff inspect all pharmaceutical companies that are licensed to manufacture vaccines and all those that have applied for licenses. Every batch of vaccine these companies make is quarantined until samples of it have been tested by the DBS; only when the manufacturer's control tests have been confirmed can the product be released. About 35,000 such tests are performed by the DBS every year.

The result of all this painstaking preparation is a small glass vial, empty except for some pinkish powder at the bottom. The vial is sealed with a cap of metal foil attached to a rubber stopper. In his office, the doctor peels off this cap, fills a syringe with a special diluting fluid, and injects it into the vial through the stopper. The powder dissolves, the fluid is drawn out through the needle, and the vaccine is ready to be injected.

It all sounds so simple. And it is, in countries where medical services are readily available and children get routine care. But in many parts of the world, preventable diseases are still a serious problem. Bringing the benefits of modern medicine to everybody everywhere is one of the great challenges of our day.

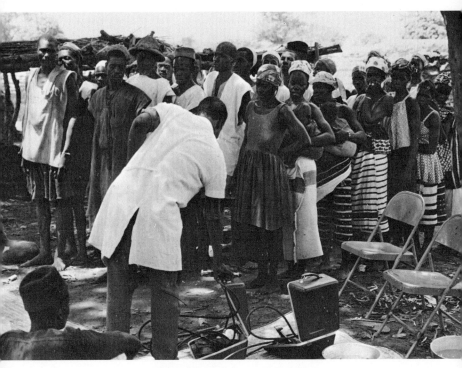

Vaccination teams try to reach every
inhabitant of this village in Mali.

9

Warding Off the Evil Wind

No more smallpox, anywhere, ever. There was a
time when that would have sounded like an impossible
dream. But in 1958, the governing body of the World
Health Organization, a specialized agency of the
United Nations, actually passed a resolution to rid
the world of smallpox. In 1967, an intensive ten-year
program was undertaken, with 1976 as the target date.

Smallpox no longer exists in countries where
children are vaccinated routinely. By 1950, Europe
and North and Central America were completely
free of it. But even though a safe, effective means of
prevention has been available for more than 150
years, smallpox still plagues parts of Asia, Africa,
and South America. Eighty thousand cases of it were
reported as recently as 1968.

It's easy enough to vaccinate people in countries
where there are modern hospitals and enough doctors
to go around, but where health services are lacking
and populations widely scattered, it can be extremely
difficult. The Republic of Mali in West Africa, for
example, has only one doctor for every 40,000 people.
And until very recently, smallpox was one of its major
health problems. In Mali, smallpox is sometimes called

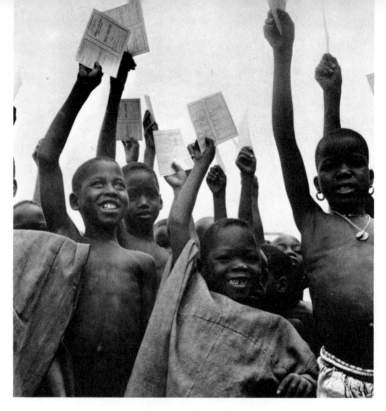

These children display their vaccination
certificates with pride.

the "evil wind," because of the way its rash reaches
every part of the body.

Mali stretches from the Sahara Desert in the north,
through semiarid country, to the grasslands, or
savanna, in the south. The Niger River flows across
the semiarid land and through part of the savanna as
well. During the rainy season, from June to October,
the Niger floods a plain about the size of the state of
Maine. Then, when the rains stop, the waters recede
again.

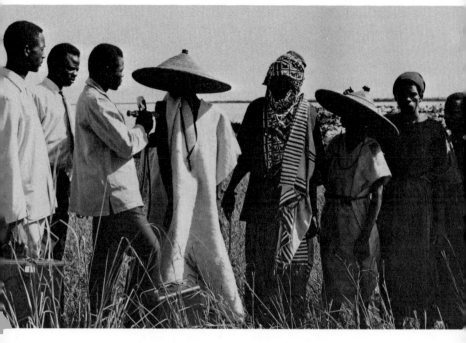

Teams must leave the village to vaccinate
the nomads on their travels.

Life in Mali revolves largely around the seasons
and the rainfall. In the Niger flood plain, nomads
travel in a seasonal orbit in search of water and
pastureland. When the river floods, they go up to the
plateau country. During the dry season, they return
to the flood plain, following the Niger until it
reaches Lake Debo. On the Niger itself, fishermen
follow the fish downstream. And in the desert, camel
nomads travel with their flocks.

It isn't easy to vaccinate people who are always on

the move this way, and for a while it seemed almost impossible to rid Mali of its smallpox. Even when most of a district's inhabitants were vaccinated, smallpox would break out there again, sometimes only a few months after the vaccinators had left. The trouble was traced to the nomads; only a small number of them were being immunized, and the rest were carrying smallpox from one village to the next.

This was the situation in 1967, when Dr. Pascal Imperato, of the United States Public Health Service, arrived to direct Mali's smallpox eradication program. Dr. Imperato has a special interest in anthropology. He made a thorough study of the nomads' paths and planned the vaccinators' routes accordingly.

Traveling by truck, on roads that were often no more than rutted lanes, the vaccinators went from village to village. They stationed themselves at the entrances to marketplaces, climbed ladders to reach settlements that were dug into the sides of cliffs, and followed fishermen down the river. In June, when the nomads arrived at Lake Debo, the vaccinators were there to meet them.

A number of technological advances made the vaccinators' work a lot easier. Freeze-dried vaccines, a recent innovation, can be carried to the most remote jungle village without danger of spoiling. And with a jet injector gun, hundreds of people can be inoculated in a very short time. The jet injector works very much the way an air rifle does. Its reservoir can hold from fifty to five hundred doses of vaccine, and these are shot right through the skin

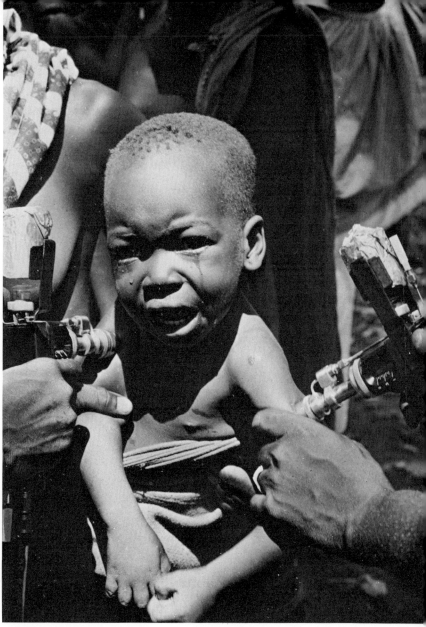

An uneasy moment: vaccination with the jet injector

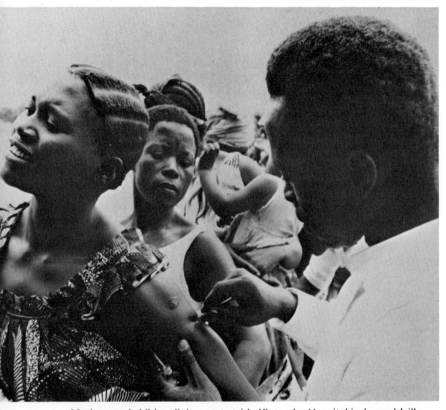

Mothers and children lining up outside Kintambo Hospital in Leopoldville, Congo, for smallpox vaccinations. In 1962, it was estimated that some 1000 residents of Leopoldville were victims of smallpox.

under high pressure. No puncture is needed, and it doesn't hurt at all. More recently, bifurcated needles have been used to vaccinate 400-500 people a day with only one-fifth the vaccine that is usually required.

Mali wasn't the only West African country to embark on a smallpox eradication program. Vaccinators were at work in eighteen others as well. With the help of the United States and the World Health Organization, these countries had set out to rid themselves of smallpox. At the same time, they hoped to control the spread of measles. The West and Central Africa Regional Smallpox Eradication and Measles Control Program was underway.

Why smallpox *eradication* but measles *control*? Measles is a highly contagious disease. It strikes nearly all African children, usually before they are two years old. Scattered over a vast area, these children can be reached only by mobile vaccination units. With large numbers of babies being born all the time, it is never possible to immunize all the susceptible children at once. Somewhere, someplace, the measles virus is bound to strike. Doctors can keep it from spreading too far, but they can never stamp it out altogether.

Smallpox, on the other hand, may soon be found only in history books. Less contagious than measles, smallpox can usually be wiped out by vaccinating 80% of a population within a period of four to five years. And that is exactly what the smallpox eradication program has done in West and Central Africa.

When the program began, American doctors trained 4000 Africans to administer vaccinations and recognize diseases. These vaccinators knew the people's customs and were able to reach large numbers of them. Under the supervision of physicians, they inoculated people of all ages against smallpox and small children against measles. In November, 1969, the 100-millionth smallpox vaccination was administered at a ceremony in Bourbon, Niger. More than five-sixths of the West and Central Africans had been vaccinated.

Results came quickly. Mali had had 1706 cases of smallpox in 1961; by 1968 the number was down to 58. Of the more than 47,000 cases the whole world had in 1969, only one occurred in Mali. In fact, by the end of August, 1969, there had been only one small outbreak of smallpox reported in all of West and Central Africa. Similar efforts had reduced the number of cases in other parts of the world as well.

Doctors must stay on guard long after the mass immunizations are over. Any cases of smallpox that do break out must be investigated quickly. From whom did the patient catch the disease? Who is likely to catch it from him? One by one, susceptible people who have had contact with a smallpox patient must be sought out and vaccinated. Infants must be vaccinated too, and so must international travelers.

Smallpox and measles aren't the only targets of the WHO's world-wide fight against virus diseases. Polio is another problem that still faces many countries. Where mass vaccination campaigns have been carried out successfully, polio has all but disappeared. But waging a successful fight against polio is easier in some parts of the world than in others.

In temperate climates, more than 90% of the
children who get live polio vaccine develop protective
antibodies. But in tropical and semitropical countries,
this same vaccine is often only half as effective. In
some parts of the world, polio is even on the rise.
This is just one of the many problems in virus diseases
that WHO researchers are trying to solve.

The World Health Organization has thirty virus
laboratories in twelve different countries. Each
concentrates on a special group of viruses. These
laboratories store different virus strains for purposes
of comparison and identification. They also train
virologists and give advice to national virus laboratories whenever they need it.

Because of its international scope, the WHO can
study the antibodies of people all over the world.
These antibodies are the tracks left behind by viruses
and other germs. By studying them, doctors can
find out where different diseases have already been
and where they are likely to turn up. National health
programs are often planned around these findings.

New vaccines are being developed with an eye to
both efficiency and economy. Research has shown
that many vaccines are just as effective in combination
as they are by themselves. Smallpox and measles
have been tried together, and so have measles,
smallpox and yellow fever, and measles, mumps and
rubella. Just one injection of these mixed vaccines
can be effective against two or three different
diseases.

When epidemics do break out, the WHO stands
ready to help. Supplies of vaccines and injectors are

kept on hand in laboratories all over the world, and teams of vaccinators are trained in advance to use them. But not all epidemics can be predicted. From time to time, new viruses appear or old ones change. When this happens, quick action and close cooperation are needed to keep the situation under control.

10

The Smartest Germ in Town

It's a small world, even for viruses. Traveling by ocean liner and jet aircraft, they can circle the globe in a matter of weeks. An epidemic that starts on one side of the world can often erupt on the other.

That's exactly what happened in the summer and fall of 1968. In mid-July of that year, an epidemic of influenza broke out in Hong Kong. By the end of the month, half a million cases had been reported there. Within two weeks the epidemic had reached Singapore; within four it had spread to Taiwan, Malaysia, Viet Nam, and the Philippines. Then it struck India, Iran, Thailand, and northern Australia. It was only a matter of time before ships carried the disease to Japan and the western coast of the United States.

In 1947, the World Health Organization had set up an influenza program to deal with just such an emergency. Now, at the WHO's National Influenza Center in Hong Kong, the virus responsible for the outbreaks was isolated. Then it was sent to two international influenza centers, one in London and one in Atlanta, Georgia, where it was tested against all existing flu vaccines. The results were alarming.

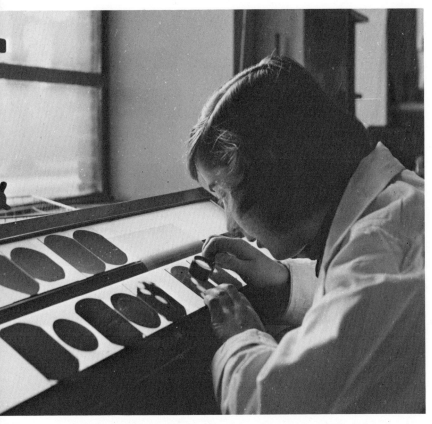
This researcher is studying electron micrographs of the influenza virus at the WHO World Influenza Reference Center in London.

Not a single one of the available vaccines offered protection against Hong Kong flu. A new vaccine, custom-tailored to the Hong Kong strain, would be needed, and quickly, if a world-wide epidemic were to be stemmed.

By mid-August, 80 national influenza laboratories in 55 countries had been informed of the appearance of the new virus strain, and samples of it had been made available to them. In the United States, the Surgeon General asked American drug companies to come to the rescue with an effective vaccine. Six of them agreed to try and meet the challenge.

In Pennsylvania, a warehouse was converted to a fully equipped biological production laboratory in just 23 days. The flu virus is grown in chick embryos, and fertile eggs are scarce at the end of the summer. Farmers all over the country were called upon to supply as many as they could. In no time at all, round-the-clock production was underway. But if man moved fast, the virus moved even faster. In October, just three weeks before the first batches of vaccine were released, Hong Kong flu broke out in Needles, a small town in southern California. Before long, it had spread from coast to coast.

This wasn't the first bout with the influenza virus, and it certainly wouldn't be the last. Influenza has been coming and going for centuries. Ancient Italian astronomers gave it its name; they thought its periodic appearances were influenced by the stars. Influenza is the Italian word for influence.

The influenza virus was isolated for the first time

in 1933 during a London epidemic, when ferrets were infected with washings from the throats of human flu victims. In both appearance and behavior, the flu virus has turned out to be one of the most remarkable of them all.

Sometimes the flu virus is shaped like a long thread, but usually it is spherical. At its center is a coiled core of RNA, surrounded by the usual protein coat. Around this coat is a fatty membrane, with spikes radiating out in all directions, something like the shell of a horse chestnut.

Most viruses stay the same year after year. The smallpox virus, for example, hasn't changed since Jenner's time. The vaccine that was used to protect you against smallpox is substantially the same as the one Jenner used on little James Phipps. Someday, it will work just as well on your great-grandchildren. But last year's flu vaccine may well be ineffective against next year's virus, and so may last year's antibodies.

There are four different types of flu virus, A, B, C and D, and all of them, especially A, are subject to sudden, unpredictable changes. Over the years, A_0, A_1, and A_2 have emerged. The Hong Kong flu virus, different from all of these, was A_2-Hong Kong-68. Major changes in the flu virus occur at intervals of about ten years, with minor ones in between. No wonder Dr. Daniel Mullally, chief of the Vaccine Development Branch of the National Institute of Allergy and Infectious Diseases, has called it "the smartest germ in town."

If the flu virus weren't able to change so frequently, it would probably die out. It has never been known to live outside the body, so its only hope for survival is to bypass the immunity that is built up against it. The types of flu virus that least match people's antibodies at any given time are the ones most likely to thrive.

All the different strains of flu virus cause the same old symptoms, although some are more virulent than others. The flu virus kills the cells in the outer layer of the respiratory tract, causing irritation which leads to sneezing and coughing. The fever, chills, and ache-all-over feeling that go with them are probably part of the body's reaction to the discharge of the breakdown products of these dying cells. The illness is usually over in three or four days, but in some people, especially the very young and the very old, it can lead to bacterial pneumonia.

The worst outbreak of influenza on record was the world-wide epidemic, or pandemic, of 1918. In fact, the Spanish flu, as it was called, was by far the greatest plague of all time. The virus that caused it was particularly deadly, and often left its victims open to the ravages of pneumonia. This was before the days of antibiotics, when pneumonia was the number one killer. During the winter of 1918-1919, twenty million deaths around the world were blamed either on influenza or the pneumonia that followed it.

No one who was alive in 1918 could forget the great pandemic. Whole families were sick, without fuel or food. People wore gauze masks on the street.

Hospitals were jammed, and nurses in short supply. So many children were orphaned in New York City that the Health Department was forced to care for them. One-fourth of all the men who died in military service during World War I were killed by the flu or its aftermath. There have been many flu epidemics since, but none to match that one.

It wasn't until 1942 that a vaccine was developed for flu. By that time, several strains of flu virus had been grown, both in hatching eggs and tissue cultures. Dr. Thomas Francis and Dr. Jonas Salk incorporated all of them into the new vaccine. When flu struck the following year, the vaccine seemed to offer good protection. Then, in 1947, the flu virus took on another of its many disguises. And against this 1947 model, the vaccine was almost completely useless.

By this time, virologists were beginning to realize that it wasn't enough to keep up with the flu virus; they had to stay one jump ahead of it. To make this possible, the World Health Organization established its network of worldwide "listening posts," where new virus strains can be identified as soon as they appear.

Public health officials still worry about the pandemic of 1918. Why was it so severe and so devastating? Is it ever likely to recur? Could anything be done to stop it if it did? If the virus that caused the pandemic could be recovered, many of these questions might be answered. Doctors once thought that the guilty germ might lie preserved, deep in the arctic, in the frozen bodies of its Eskimo victims.

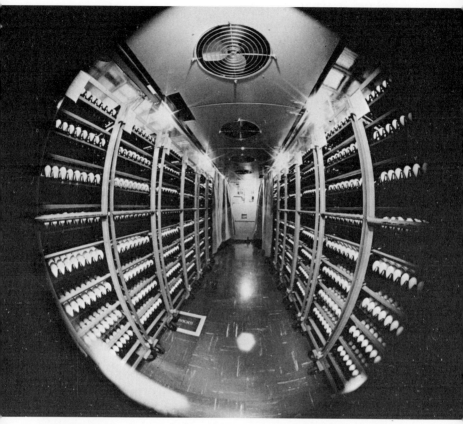

Large incubators, each capable of holding 46,000 eggs, were used for vaccine production during the race to prevent an epidemic of influenza in 1968.

In 1951, an expedition, unique in medical history, set out to try to recover it.

The 1918 flu pandemic reached Alaska in November of that year via an Army transport bound from Seattle to Nome. Flu was raging in Seattle when the transport left, and many of the passengers became ill en route. Once in Nome, they were cared for by Eskimo women, and within days large numbers of Eskimos took sick and died. Many were buried in "permafrost" areas, where the deeper layers of earth are always frozen. One of the victims, George Prosser, was known to be buried near Nome, and the project became known as Operation George.

After a number of false starts, the investigators of Operation George found several well-preserved bodies of Alaskan flu victims buried in a tundra slope in Golovin. Samples of lung and other tissues were removed from them, sealed in sterile jars, and delivered, frozen, to Harvard University, the University of Michigan, and the U.S. Army Medical Service Graduate School.

Laboratory workers at these institutions tried every trick they knew to find flu virus in these tissue samples. They inoculated ferrets with them, hoping to pass the infection on. Using hatching eggs, they tried to grow the virus. They injected rabbits with the material and tested them for flu antibodies. In no case were positive results obtained. For reasons unknown, the flu virus had failed to survive in the frozen tissue.

With the failure of Operation George, doctors lost

their last chance to discover exactly what caused the 1918 pandemic. There have been two pandemics since then, Asian flu in 1957 and Hong Kong flu in 1968, but neither was nearly as severe. However, there is reason to think that we may not be so lucky in the future.

When Asian flu hit in 1957, a Dutch doctor discovered that some elderly residents of the Netherlands, people in their seventies at the time, had antibodies against it. Some Americans of the same age did too. Among other age groups, no such antibodies could be found. The same thing happened when Hong Kong flu struck in 1968; a few people in their seventies were the only ones who had natural immunity to it. This seems to suggest that the different types of flu virus appear in cycles of seventy years. If this proves to be the case, there might be another severe pandemic around 1988. By then, however, there may be better methods for dealing with it.

Most doctors are dissatisfied with the present means of fighting flu, and a great deal of research is aimed at improving them. One of the most promising approaches is based on what virologists have come to call "original antigenic sin."

When a child has his first bout with flu, he develops antibodies against the particular type of virus that attacks him. Later, if he encounters another type of flu virus, he develops a new type of antibodies, but he also develops more of the ones he already has. This process continues throughout his life. For reasons not yet understood, a person's first exposure to the

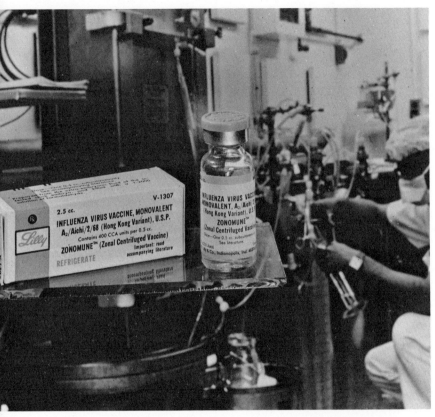

With the combined efforts of the WHO, government agencies and vaccine manufacturers, a new flu vaccine was produced against the Hong Kong strain.

flu virus has a lifelong effect on his antibody pattern.

If children were given a vaccine containing all the major types of flu virus, each exposure to flu would strengthen their broad natural resistance. Until recently, such a vaccine would have produced serious side effects. Now, with new methods of purification, it may soon become a reality.

11

German Measles:
A Threat to the Unborn

Thirteen blind babies. That was the number that Dr. Norman Gregg, an Australian ophthalmologist, saw in 1941. The babies all had cataracts, opaque defects in the lenses of their eyes. And the cataracts were congenital; the babies had been born with them. Concerned at seeing so many infants with such a rare condition, Dr. Gregg questioned other ophthalmologists in nearby communities. He was astounded to learn of 65 other cases of congenital cataracts, a total of 78.

Delving further, Dr. Gregg discovered that the 78 babies had a number of other symptoms in common. Most of them were quite small, ill-nourished, and difficult to feed. Many had congenital heart disease. Dr. Gregg was struck by the fact that all had been born six or seven months after a large epidemic of German measles. Most striking of all, 68 of the 78 mothers remembered having had German measles during the first few months of their pregnancies.

German measles is a mild disease, so mild, in fact, that it wasn't recognized until 1815. That was when an English doctor, William Maton, first described it. Widespread epidemics had occurred in Germany, where the disease was called *rötheln* to distinguish it from regular measles, or rubeola. English-speaking people found *"rötheln"* hard to pronounce, so they called it German measles, or rubella.

Until 1941, rubella wasn't much cause for concern. A pinkish-red rash, a few swollen glands, and it was over, usually in about three· days. There was no fever, and the patient didn't feel particularly sick. Doctors could never be quite sure whether a mild illness with a rash was rubella or one of a number of similar diseases. But once they learned to recognize the symptoms of rubella in the newborn child, there was no mistaking it.

John Kenny was a typical rubella baby. The youngest of four boys, he lives with his family in Hicksville, New York. About eight months before John was born, one of his brothers invited a neighborhood friend in to play. The friend seemed perfectly healthy at the time, but the next day he broke out in a rash. The diagnosis: German measles.

Aware of the threat to her unborn child, Mrs. Kenny sought medical help at once. She was given gamma globulin, in the hope that it would prevent her baby from developing birth defects. But gamma globulin rarely helps where German measles is concerned. Two weeks later, Mrs. Kenny broke out in the rash herself. And when her baby was born, it was clear that he had been infected too.

John was what doctors call a "blueberry muffin baby." He was covered with bluish-red spots, a sign that his blood platelets were deficient. At birth he weighed a scant five and a half pounds. Both his liver and his spleen were enlarged, and his eyes looked as though someone had sprinkled salt and pepper deep inside them. This common sign of congenital rubella is caused by a clumping of the pigment in the retina. Fortunately, it does not interfere with vision.

Babies like John can shed rubella virus from their noses and throats for many months, sometimes for as long as two years. Before long, the virus spread by John was responsible for two new cases of German measles in the Kenny household.

When John was three months old, he left some applesauce in his dish, and two of his brothers finished it up for him. Neither boy had caught German measles from the neighborhood friend who had given it to their mother, from their mother herself, or, up to this time, from John, but now, within two weeks, both of them came down with it.

German measles is peculiar this way; its spread is thoroughly unpredictable. Less contagious than the other childhood diseases, it fails to infect about one child in five. This means that many women, like Mrs. Kenny, are in danger of catching German measles and passing it on to their unborn children.

As John grew older, the bluish-red spots faded and his liver and spleen returned to normal size. At the same time, signs of permanent damage began to show up. At an age when normal children are beginning to walk, John couldn't pull himself up to a sitting position. He didn't develop speech either, or respond to requests from his mother. Tests showed that he had spastic cerebral palsy and a severe hearing loss.

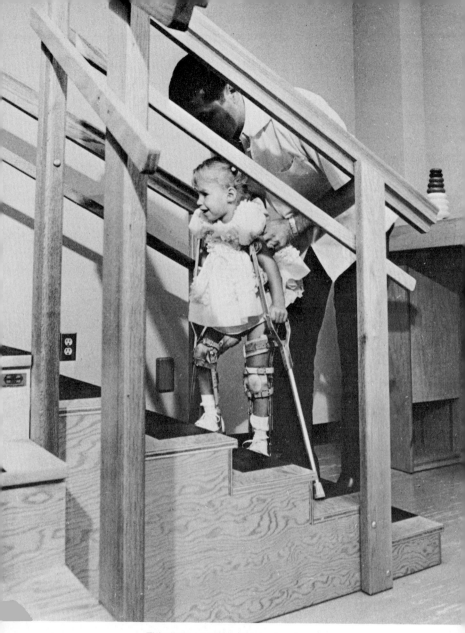

This little girl has cerebral palsy,
one of the disorders caused by the
rubella virus.

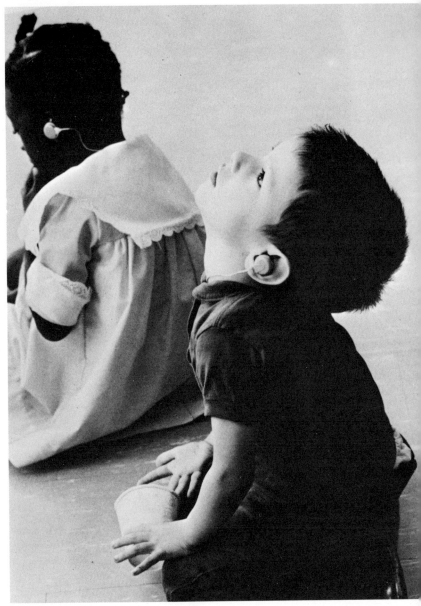

Hearing loss and mental retardation are also common in children whose mothers had rubella in pregnancy.

The rubella virus infects every part of the unborn child, but it has four special targets: the heart, the brain, the ears, and the eyes. In John's case, the part of the brain that controls the muscles was injured, making it impossible for him to straighten his legs or flatten his feet. Damage to his inner ear had left him partially deaf.

John had some heart damage too, a murmur caused by a narrowing of his main pulmonary arteries. The rubella virus prevents cells from dividing normally. If these cells are in the developing blood vessels of an unborn child, constrictions can result. Many rubella babies have a more serious heart condition, *patent ductus arteriosus*, which can only be corrected with open heart surgery.

A number of different specialists are needed to treat children like John Kenny. Rubella clinics commonly employ pediatricians, cardiologists, specialists in rehabilitation medicine, otologists, audiologists, teachers of the deaf, physical therapists, social workers, bracemakers, and psychologists. John has received the help of many of them.

Today John walks with braces and crutches, but he may one day learn to do without them. He attends a school for the deaf, where he is being taught to speak and to understand others. John's hearing loss is considerable. With a hearing aid, he can hear a dog bark or a phone ring. He turns around at the sound of a voice, but he doesn't understand words in the normal way.

Children like John often have language problems that go far beyond their hearing deficiencies. Sometimes they hear sounds but are unable to decode them. Since they don't understand what they hear, they have trouble learning to speak. The child with a hearing loss or a language impairment needs years of special schooling that must start when he is very young.

As soon as doctors realized how severely German measles can damage babies like John Kenny, they took a long second look at it. What had seemed to be a mild disease suddenly became a major health problem. Research programs were established all over the world to learn more about the rubella birth defect problem and to find ways to control and prevent German measles. Most doctors thought that German measles was a viral disease, and the first order of business was to isolate the virus in the laboratory.

For twenty years doctors tried and failed to isolate the virus that causes German measles. While other viruses were trapped and tamed in rapid succession, the German measles virus stubbornly refused to grow. Then, in 1961, two events occurred which finally led to its capture.

In Boston, a ten-year-old boy developed an illness that seemed to be an unusually bad case of German measles. The rash and the swollen glands were typical, but the boy was much sicker than the usual German measles patient, and he had a high fever. His father was very concerned about him.

The concerned father in this case was Dr. Thomas Weller, the Nobel Prize-winning virologist. Dr. Weller's son recovered uneventfully, but not before his father had taken a specimen of urine to his

Harvard laboratory and added it to some tissue cultures of human skin and muscle cells. Dr. Weller watched the cultures for six weeks, but nothing seemed to happen to them. Undaunted, he passed the fluids from these cultures into cultures of human amnion cells. Four weeks later his efforts were rewarded. There were changes in these new cultures that clearly indicated the presence of a virus.

In the meantime, at Fort Dix in New Jersey, an outbreak of German measles was spreading rapidly through the battalions. A team of virologists from the Walter Reed Army Medical Center seized the opportunity to take throat swabbings and blood specimens from the infected men. These were inoculated into cultures of African green monkey kidney (AGMK) cells. The cultures were examined carefully each day, but no changes could be detected in them. However, instead of writing this off as another failure in the long search for the rubella virus, the virologists at Walter Reed decided to apply a technique developed in England the year before.

At the Common Cold Research Unit in Salisbury, Dr. D.A.J. Tyrrell and his co-workers had been trying to isolate rhinoviruses, an important cause of the common cold. They had found that certain rhinoviruses could infect AGMK cells without having any visible effect on them. To prove that the rhinovirus was really there, they added a second virus, echovirus, to the same cultures. Normally, echovirus infects AGMK cells rapidly, producing visible signs of damage. But in cells already infected with rhino-

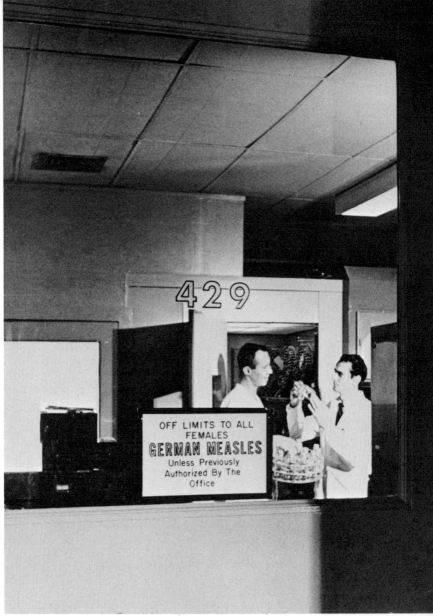

Before the German measles vaccine, certain laboratories were off limits to women.

virus, no such signs appeared. The first infection was somehow able to prevent the second one. This is called viral interference.

The workers at Walter Reed now added echovirus to the cultures they had tried to infect with rubella. For purposes of comparison, they also added it to some uninoculated cultures. The results were striking. Within two days the uninoculated cultures were full of holes. Many of their cells were dying, leaving spaces in what had been a smooth, tightly packed sheet. But the first group of cultures looked exactly the way they had before. The rubella virus was there all right, preventing the echovirus from infecting and destroying the cells.

Now the workers at Harvard and at Walter Reed joined forces. They compared the viruses they had isolated and found that they were one and the same. In an outstanding example of scientific cooperation, the two discoveries were reported side by side in the same medical journal. The rubella virus had finally been captured, and it was hoped that a vaccine could soon be developed.

For the vaccine makers, rubella is in a class by itself. Measles and polio are serious diseases. They can cause prolonged illness, even death. The rubella virus, on the other hand, produces a mild illness in both children and adults; its only real threat is to the embryo developing inside its mother.

A rubella vaccine was needed to safeguard unborn children by protecting their mothers. But vaccinating pregnant women against rubella could be dangerous. Suppose the vaccine itself caused birth defects.

There was no way to find out whether it would or not without actually trying it out, and this was impossible because of the tremendous risk involved.

In view of these problems, an alternate approach was chosen. Most women, like Mrs. Kenny, catch rubella from children. Protecting children from rubella would protect expectant mothers too, without any risk to their babies. It was decided to develop a vaccine that could be given to children and to young women before they had babies. Such a vaccine would have to produce the same lasting immunity as natural rubella without any of the symptoms. In addition, it would have to be non-contagious. There must be no danger of vaccinated children spreading the vaccine virus to pregnant women.

A number of investigators set out to tame the rubella virus. One of them was Dr. Paul Parkman, a member of the team that had first isolated it at Walter Reed. Completing his army service, Dr. Parkman moved his laboratory to the Division of Biologics Standards (DBS) of the National Institutes of Health. There, he and Dr. Harry Meyer started the rubella virus on a long series of passages through tissue cultures of African green monkey cells. At regular intervals, they compared the passaged virus with its unattenuated parent.

There were 77 passages in all. The resulting virus was called a high passage virus, HPV-77 for short, and laboratory tests showed that it was very different from the natural rubella virus. Its effect on rabbit kidney cells was far more destructive. And in rhesus monkeys it produced no contagious disease at all. Monkeys inoculated with natural rubella virus develop a mild infection and pass it on to their cage-mates.

It was time to test the new vaccine on human volunteers. The investigators chose a residential school in Arkansas, The Arkansas Children's Colony, where small groups of children live in separate cottages. The school was isolated from the community, so there was no danger of contagion from the vaccinated children. And since the children lived at the school, they were available for constant medical supervision. Sixteen families agreed to let their daughters participate in the first trials.

Drs. Parkman and Meyer arrived at the colony in October, 1965, with specimens of HPV-77 packed in dry ice. Eight of the girls were inoculated with the vaccine, and eight others served as controls to determine whether or not the virus would spread through the group. For two months these sixteen girls were isolated from the rest of the school. Throat swabs and blood specimens were taken from each of them every day to check for infection and to make sure that the girls who had been inoculated were developing antibodies against rubella.

When the experiment was over, the doctors had just the results they had hoped for. None of the vaccinated children became ill, but all of them developed antibodies against the rubella virus. The unvaccinated children were completely unaffected.

This small trial was followed by larger ones, and when the vaccine had been thoroughly tested it was made available to research scientists in commercial

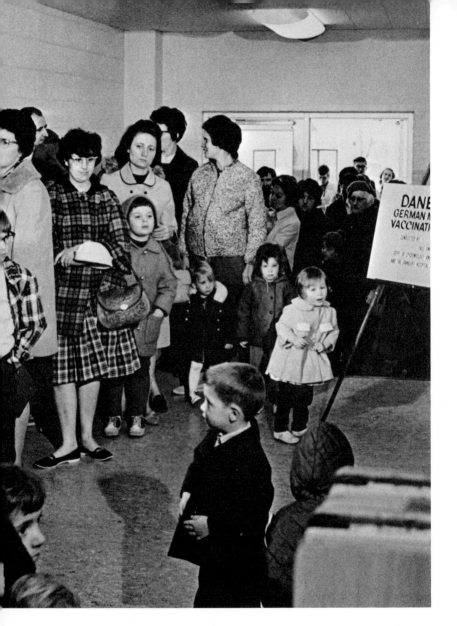

A German measles vaccination clinic.

pharmaceutical companies. By June, 1969, the first rubella vaccine was licensed in the United States. It was made from the HPV-77 strain, but two other strains of rubella vaccine have also been developed. Only time will tell which one is best.

Getting a vaccine to the people who need it is always a problem, and with rubella the job is especially difficult. Parents must be made to understand that the rubella virus causes birth defects and that children who are not inoculated against it may one day be a source of infection to expectant mothers. Newspapers, radio, television and loudspeaker trucks are used to get this message to as many people as possible, and free rubella vaccinations are made available to all who need them.

Epidemics of German measles occur at intervals of seven to ten years. The last one, in 1964, probably affected more than 120,000 pregnant women, about 40,000 of them in the critical early months. At least 30,000 rubella babies were born after that single epidemic. Now, with a rubella vaccine available, there is every reason to hope that the rubella epidemic of 1964 will be the last one in medical history.

12

Hepatitis: The Doctors' Dilemma

It was August, 1969. The football fans were still on vacation, but at campuses all over the country the teams were back for pre-season practice. One of those teams was never to have a football season that year. A virus would see to that.

At Holy Cross College in Worcester, Massachusetts, the practice went well at first, with only the expected number of sprains and bruises. But as the team got ready for its first game, other problems began to arise. Some of the players lost their appetites and began feeling weak and tired. Several were feverish and noticed that their urine was much darker than usual. A few developed stomach aches. Then some of the sick players became jaundiced. Their skin turned yellow, and so did the whites of their eyes. By this time, the college doctor knew he was dealing with an outbreak of hepatitis.

Epidemics of hepatitis often occur in groups that live and work closely together. The disease affects fighting men so often that military surgeons were the first to describe it. Napoleon's forces were weakened by hepatitis during their unsuccessful Egyptian campaign. Hepatitis was a problem during the Civil War too, and during World War I. But it was a tragic accident in the second World War that brought about the first real progress in understanding this perplexing disease.

In 1942, yellow fever vaccine was given routinely to all U.S. servicemen, and with it came a sharp increase in the Army's hepatitis problem. Soldiers were getting hepatitis by the thousands, usually three or four months after their yellow fever inoculations. The trouble was traced to the human blood serum in which the vaccine virus was then suspended. Unknown to the vaccine-makers, some of the donors of this serum had had hepatitis, and the infectious agent was still in their blood. Unwittingly, the doctors had passed it on.

Spurred on by this discovery, investigators made a number of others. Hepatitis is caused by a filterable particle, presumably a virus. It is widespread in the civilian population as well as in the military. In fact, most of its victims are children under fifteen.

Like polio, hepatitis is usually a mild infection, especially in young people. Often it goes completely unnoticed. Sometimes it just causes fatigue, nausea, fever, and headache, the symptoms that characterize so many other virus diseases. But the hepatitis virus has a particular liking for liver cells. That is how it got its name; hepatitis is Latin for "inflammation of the liver." When the hepatitis virus infects the liver cells, they swell, blocking the flow of bile. The bile accumulates in the bloodstream and turns the victim yellow with jaundice. Liver cells have a remarkable capacity to restore themselves, and most patients recover from hepatitis in a matter of weeks or months. In rare cases, though, the damage to the liver can be fatal.

There are two forms of hepatitis. Infectious hepatitis, the kind the football players had, is spread from one person to another or picked up from contaminated food or water. Clams and oysters can be a source of hepatitis if they are harvested from polluted water. Hepatitis has also been spread by custards, smoked meats, and gravies. In the case of the football players, the source of infection turned out to be a contaminated water supply in their locker room.

Serum hepatitis is usually spread by doctors themselves. This is the kind that the soldiers got along with their yellow fever vaccine. In the past, it was often caused by contaminated hypodermic or tattoo needles.

Tattooing is done by sticking a needle just under the skin. If this needle is used on a person incubating hepatitis, it can transmit the infection to many others. Tattooing parlors have now been outlawed in the United States, and today this mode of spread is rare. Disposable needles and syringes, which are used only once, have decreased the chances of getting hepatitis from contaminated medical instruments. But for the person in need of a blood transfusion, serum hepatitis is still a special problem.

Many people have hepatitis without knowing it. Afterward, they can carry the virus in their blood for five years, or even longer. With six million blood transfusions being given in America each year, some are bound to carry the hepatitis virus. There is no way to kill the virus without destroying the usefulness of the blood at the same time.

Doctors try to minimize the danger of serum hepatitis by giving blood transfusions only when they are absolutely necessary. They have stopped using "pooled" blood plasma, plasma taken from many donors and mixed together, because of the greater risk it carries. But transfusions are still a frequent cause of hepatitis. The number of cases of serum hepatitis may even be on the rise.

Serum hepatitis causes all the same symptoms that infectious hepatitis does. The only real difference between them is the time they take to develop. Infectious hepatitis takes two to six weeks; serum hepatitis takes several months. It isn't unusual for people to find themselves turning yellow long after they have recovered from surgical operations.

Hepatitis is one of the great puzzles of modern virology. The same investigators who have conquered polio and won global races with influenza are completely baffled by it. They have never been able to grow the guilty virus or to see it in an electron microscope. No laboratory animal has been found to be susceptible to it. But even though a hepatitis vaccine is a long way off, several other methods of prevention have been developed.

Gamma globulin, once used to protect children against measles, is also useful in preventing hepatitis, and for the very same reason. Hepatitis, like measles, is a disease that most people have at some time in their lives, and gamma globulin is rich in hepatitis antibodies. Dr. Joseph Stokes, of the University of Pennsylvania, was able to show that these antibodies can often prevent hepatitis, or at least decrease its severity.

In the summer of 1944, a hepatitis epidemic broke out in a children's camp. Dr. Stokes immediately treated 53 of the healthy campers with gamma globulin. The remaining 278 were untreated. Only 11 of the treated children developed hepatitis, and of these only 3 had jaundice. But 185 of the untreated children got hepatitis, 125 with jaundice. Without gamma globulin, the chances of getting hepatitis were more than three times as great and the cases that did develop were more severe.

It was also interesting to note that the treated children who did get hepatitis got it within ten days of their gamma globulin injections. Since hepatitis takes more than ten days to develop, these children must have been infected before the antibodies in the gamma globulin had a chance to go to work. Given before the infection began, the gamma globulin seemed to offer complete protection.

Dr. Stokes' findings were confirmed by many other investigators, and ever since then people who have been exposed to hepatitis, or who expect to be exposed, have been treated with gamma globulin. Dr. Stokes received the Medal of Freedom from the U.S. Government for his important contribution to the control of hepatitis.

Until recently, gamma globulin was effective only in preventing infectious hepatitis. Against serum hepatitis, it was almost useless. But a recent discovery has made it possible to prevent serum hepatitis too, with gamma globulin of a very special kind.

The clue came from a most unlikely source: an Australian aborigine. While comparing blood samples from people all over the world, Dr. Baruch S. Blumberg and his colleagues at the Institute for Cancer Research in Philadelphia were struck by the fact that an antibody in a New Yorker's blood serum reacted with an antigen in the blood of an aborigine. The doctors called it "Australia antigen."

Other blood samples were tested for Australia antigen, and thousands of people were found to have it. Victims of leukemia had it in unusually large numbers, and so did mongoloid children. But as the study progressed, it became clear that patients with serum hepatitis were the most regular and reliable carriers of Australia antigen.

There was further evidence to link Australia antigen and serum hepatitis. People who received transfusions of blood containing Australia antigen regularly came down with hepatitis. So did people whose negative antigen tests suddenly turned positive. In fact, Australia antigen was so closely related to hepatitis that its name was changed to hepatitis associated antigen, or HAA.

Antibodies to HAA are rarely found in the blood of normal people. But one group of patients, those with hemophilia, have an abundance of these antibodies in their serum. People with hemophilia need hundreds of blood transfusions to stay alive, and they are often exposed to blood containing HAA. From the plasma of one of them, Dr. Alfred M. Prince, of the New York Blood Center, prepared some gamma globulin that was unusually rich in HAA antibodies.

Dr. Saul Krugman and Dr. Joan Giles, both of the New York University Medical Center, were able

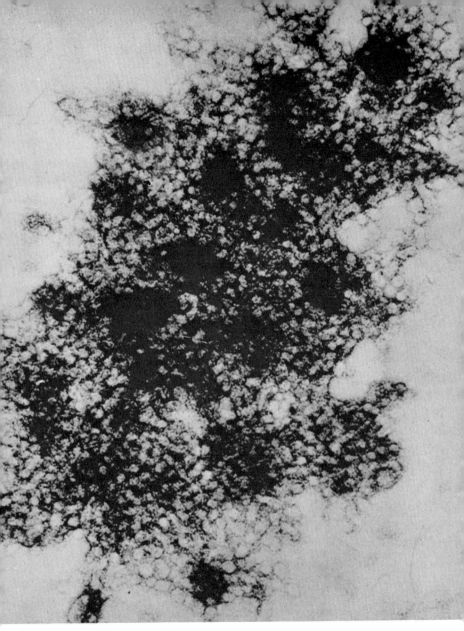

The discovery of this hepatitis associated antigen, here photographed with the electron microscope, provided the first major breakthrough in the fight against serum hepatitis.

to show that this special gamma globulin gave excellent protection against serum hepatitis. First they exposed fifteen children to blood containing HAA. Four hours later, five of the children were given regular gamma globulin while the other ten got gamma globulin from the hemophiliac. The regular gamma globulin failed to protect three of the five children who received it, but all ten in the other group were fully protected.

This was passive immunization, the injection of ready-made antibodies from another person. Dr. Krugman's team was also able to give children active immunization agents against serum hepatitis by stimulating them to produce their own antibodies. To do this they used a vaccine made from HAA that had been boiled for one minute.

Doctors have developed a quick, efficient test for HAA in the blood of prospective donors. Antibodies for HAA are added to a drop of the donor's blood serum. If HAA is present, a characteristic precipitate forms. The test isn't sensitive enough to detect HAA in very small amounts, but its widespread use should reduce the risk of serum hepatitis considerably.

Just what exactly is HAA? Chances are that it is a virus, or at least a portion of one. In both size and shape, it is similar to many known virus particles. Under the electron microscope, HAA appears to be a spherical particle, sometimes with a central core, sometimes without one. So far, it has refused to grow either in tissue cultures or laboratory animals.

The results that have been obtained in immunizing children against serum hepatitis are promising, but they are still very preliminary. A number of years will probably be needed to develop and evaluate a successful vaccine. Hepatitis is just one of the many viral diseases that will continue to plague us for some time to come.

13

The All Too Common Cold

Most children have seven or eight colds a year, with two-thirds of all school absences caused by colds and cold-like illnesses. Adults don't fare much better. The cost of the common cold in lost wages, lost production, and medical expenses is estimated at five billion dollars a year.

Many cold victims bundle into bed and try to relieve their discomfort. But what "goes with a cold in the nose"? Very little really. Most medications simply relieve the symptoms while nature takes its course. Few if any are aimed at the cause of the trouble. For while successful battles have been waged against such serious illnesses as yellow fever, polio, and measles, the common cold has been puzzling scientists the world over.

The cause of colds has been known since 1914. During that year, four members of Dr. Walther Kruse's laboratory staff at the Hygenic Institute of the University of Liepzig had colds all at once, and they weren't any accident. Several days earlier, when another assistant caught a cold, Dr. Kruse had passed his nasal washings through a filter and dropped them into the noses of twelve other people. When four of them came down with colds, he knew that a virus was causing them.

For nearly fifty years, scientists searched for "the cold virus." They injected infectious nasal washings into tissue cultures, but the virus mysteriously disappeared. On the rare occasions when it did grow, results were inconsistent.

Then, in 1948, the Enders team developed reliable methods for growing viruses in test tubes. For the first time, it was possible to trap viruses from the nose and throat washings of people with colds. When these were studied and compared, it became clear that colds were not caused by a single virus or even by a few different virus types. There were many families of cold viruses, some with thirty members or more.

Virus families are classified according to their chemical properties and the kind of cells they grow in. Adenoviruses, the first to be discovered, were found in human adenoid tissue. The adenoids, like the tonsils, are soft, spongy patches of lymphoid tissue. They are found above the tonsils at the back of the nose. In some children, the tonsils and adenoids become enlarged and have to be removed. "T and A's," the doctors' shorthand for tonsillectomies and adenoidectomies, are performed every day in most hospitals. These operations provide a ready source of human cells for tissue cultures.

In 1953, workers at the National Institutes of Health were growing tissue cultures of adenoidal cells. These cells grew readily in a test tube, at least at first. Then, after a few weeks, they began to degenerate. The degeneration was caused by a virus that made its home in the adenoids. More than thirty such viruses have been found, often in connection with sore throats, fevers, and eye infections. Although common in adults, these adenoviruses cause the most trouble in children and in military recruits.

From two little boys in the town of Coxsackie, New York, came a strange virus that caused a disease something like polio. It turned out to be the first of more than thirty Coxsackie viruses. Other members of this family cause sore throats, fevers, and chest pains. One is often responsible for the common cold. Coxsackie viruses are part of a larger group, the enteriviruses, that live in the human intestine. ECHO viruses belong to this group too, and they can also produce cold-like symptoms.

The parade of cold viruses doesn't stop here. Myxoviruses are also responsible for respiratory illnesses. The influenza viruses belong to this group, and so do the four para-influenza viruses that cause croup in children and colds and sore throats in adults. Another myxovirus, the respiratory syncytial or RS virus, is the most common cause of severe viral respiratory infection in infants and small children.

Important as these viruses are, the real breakthrough in cold virus research came in 1960 at the Common Cold Research Unit in Salisbury, England. When Dr. D.A.J. Tyrrell and Sir Christopher Andrewes took nasal secretions from cold patients and inoculated them into tissue cultures of African green monkey cells, they found that they had discovered a brand-new family of viruses. Called rhino, or nose, viruses, they turned out to be responsible for one-fourth to one-third of all colds. There are so many different types of rhinovirus that nobody bothers to name them; instead they are simply numbered. More than eighty of them are already known.

Dealing with so many cold viruses is difficult enough, but to make matters worse no convenient laboratory animal is susceptible to most of them. Mice, rats, guinea pigs, cotton rats, voles, hamsters, gray squirrels, hedgehogs, ferrets, pigs, chicks, and several types of monkeys have been injected with infectious nasal washings, but all in vain. Only chimpanzees get human colds, and they are scarce and expensive. As a result, people have been the guinea pigs in most of the experiments carried out on the common cold.

At the Common Cold Research Unit in Salisbury, thousands of people have allowed themselves to be exposed to colds and infected with a wide variety of cold-producing agents. Afterward, some of them have stood in a cold room with a wet bathing suit on for half an hour at a time. All of this has been part of an effort to learn more about how colds begin and how they are spread.

Some of the findings have been surprising. People worry a lot about catching colds, but research has shown that they aren't particularly contagious. Chilling doesn't seem to cause colds either. There *are* more colds in the winter, but this is probably because colds have a better chance to spread when people are crowded together indoors. Dry, heated indoor air in combination with the cold air out of doors may also make people more susceptible to colds by damaging their nasal mucosa. It is also possible that some people carry latent cold viruses that are activated by sudden changes in the weather.

Colds come back again and again because, unlike other virus infections, they don't produce lasting immunity against the germs that cause them. Instead of passing through the bloodstream as most viruses do, cold viruses infect the cells that line the respiratory tract. The antibodies produced by these cells don't last as long as antibodies that circulate in the blood.

Even if cold viruses did produce lasting immunity, it is very unlikely that they could all be combined in a single vaccine. There are just too many of them. Protecting people of all ages against colds all year round would mean immunizing them against more then one hundred different viruses.

At least one successful cold vaccine has been produced, but it is aimed only at a particular group of viruses. A killed virus vaccine was made for several types of adenovirus that cause most of the respiratory illness among military recruits. Given to the rookies at Fort Dix in 1956, it was 83% effective in keeping them off the sick list.

Similar vaccines could be developed for other special purposes. A vaccine to protect children against the RS virus, for example, is well within the realm of possibility. If just a few of the rhinoviruses turn out to be responsible for most adult colds, a vaccine could be made against them too. But vaccines like these would have limited targets. Broad protection against respiratory infections will have to come from another source.

14

Another Way to Fight Viruses

As powerful as they are, vaccines have their limitations. For illnesses that are caused by one stable virus, vaccines provide surefire protection. Even polio, which is caused by three viruses, can be prevented by vaccination. But when more than a hundred different viruses cause the same set of symptoms, as they do in the case of the common cold, vaccines are impractical. And when viruses are subject to change, as the influenza virus is, vaccines aren't always reliable.

Fortunately, antibodies aren't our only weapon against viruses. Early in the 1950's, it was discovered that some people have no antibodies at all. They have a rare disease called hypogammaglobulinemia, an inability to manufacture gamma globulin. Until the discovery of antibiotics, such people died early from bacterial infections. Now, with wonder drugs and gamma globulin to protect them, they are living to get viral infections as well. This gives doctors a chance to find out how viruses behave when there are no antibodies to neutralize them.

Surprisingly enough, people with hypogamma-globulinemia respond to viruses very much the way normal people do. They don't get any sicker than the rest of us, and they recover in the normal length of time. Something besides antibodies must be there to protect them. Doctors were anxious to discover what this "something" was and how it worked, because they hoped it would lead them to new ways of preventing virus diseases.

An important clue was found in the fact that two viruses almost never strike in the same place at once. Children rarely get measles and mumps at the same time. Monkeys with Rift Valley fever don't get yellow fever, a disease that would otherwise kill them. Somehow or other, the first virus interferes with the second one and prevents the infection it causes. This virus interference can't be due to antibodies, because two viruses can interfere even though their antibodies are very different.

The cause of virus interference was discovered in 1957 by Alick Isaacs and Jean Lindenmann at the National Institute for Medical Research in England. They found that when cells in tissue culture were infected with a virus, the culture medium changed in a remarkable way. Used to nourish fresh cells, it was able to protect them against a broad range of virus infections. There was something in the medium that prevented viruses from multiplying inside the cells. When this protective substance was isolated, it turned out to be a small protein molecule. The investigators called it interferon.

The interferon in this experiment had been manufactured by the original tissue in response to the virus that infected it. Further investigation showed that most animal cells produced interferon in response to viruses and a number of other foreign substances. And this interferon, once there was enough of it, would protect neighboring cells against any virus at all.

Interferon production, like the immune response, is part of our natural system of defense against viruses. Interferon has been detected in human blood serum during many virus infections and in other body fluids and tissues as well. To learn more about the role interferon plays in fighting off viruses, Isaacs and Lindenmann infected mice with influenza virus and tested them each day for both interferon and antibodies. At first, the virus concentration built up and so did the concentration of interferon. By the third day, both had reached their peaks. Then the virus concentration began to decrease, but the concentration of interferon remained high until the fifth day. It wasn't until a week after the mice had been infected with the virus that antibodies could be detected in their bloodstreams.

A similar response has been observed in people. When fifteen men were injected with yellow fever vaccine, interferon was detected in the blood serum of ten of them. This interferon reached its peak concentration on the sixth day after the injection, twenty-four hours before any yellow fever antibodies appeared. All this evidence suggests that interferon is an immediate, natural response to virus infection. Its effect is short-lived, but that doesn't matter; its main function is to fight off the virus until antibodies have had a chance to develop.

Interferon prepared in the laboratory can stave off viruses too. Sprayed in the nose, it prevents respiratory infections. Injected under the skin, it prevents infection by the cowpox virus. Interferon can be used over and over again without losing its effectiveness. It isn't easily destroyed by heat or chemicals; in fact, it can be stored at low temperatures and even freeze-dried. It seems to be an ideal virus-fighter. If it were available in large enough quantities, it might put an end to virus disease.

Unfortunately, using interferon to prevent virus infections isn't as easy as it might seem. The number of cells in the human body has been estimated at 10^{13}. (That's a one with thirteen zeros after it.) If hatching eggs could be used to make interferon for people, 2000 of them would be needed to make a single dose. And this dose would be effective for just a few days at the most.

But the problem is even more difficult than that. Interferon is not a single protein, but a whole family of proteins. Each animal species has an interferon all its own. Interferon produced in hen's eggs protects chick cell cultures, but not cultures of mouse cells or human cells. To be effective in people, interferon would have to be produced in a human cell culture system, and such a system is not available.

Luckily, there may be another approach. Lacking the ability to supply interferon from the outside, investigators have begun to study the way cells make interferon of their own. Once this process is understood, it may be possible to take advantage of it, just as vaccines take advantage of the body's ability to manufacture antibodies.

It was clear from the beginning that interferon doesn't damage viruses the way chemicals like formaldehyde do. Instead, it does its work inside the infected cell. A complicated series of experiments has provided some idea of the role interferon plays in preventing virus infections.

When an RNA virus enters a cell and prepares to multiply inside it, the viral RNA splits into two identical parts. RNA is usually a long, coiled strand, but when it splits this strand is doubled. The double-stranded RNA causes an "alert reaction" which stimulates the production of interferon by the infected cell. Diffusing outward, this interferon enters healthy cells and triggers the production of a protein which makes it impossible for viruses to take over the cells' machinery.

It has been found that any double-stranded RNA can trigger this "alert reaction," even if it doesn't come from a virus. Cells in tissue culture have been tested with a number of double-stranded RNA's, some naturally occurring, others laboratory produced. All share the property of inducing the cells to produce interferon.

One of these interferon inducers, Poly I:C, already has been tried on human volunteers in the form of nose drops. When challenged with rhinovirus, many of these volunteers failed to develop colds. The day may not be far off when a nasal spray will cure colds before they have a chance to develop.

15

Runaway Cells

What headline would you most like to see in your daily paper? People all over the world were asked that question, and the answer most of them gave was CANCER CURE FOUND. For the fear it inspires and the suffering it causes, no other disease can match cancer.

Healthy cells know when to stop growing. In an embryo, cells multiply very rapidly. During early life, this growth tapers off slowly, and in the adult it stops completely. The cells replenish themselves, but their total number remains the same.

Cells in tissue cultures behave much the same way. When a closed sheet of cells has been formed, with every cell touching its neighbors, the cells stop multiplying. This is known as contact inhibition.

In cancer, cells lose this ability to regulate their growth. They multiply without limit, invading normal cells and preventing them from functioning. When an organism has cancer, all its energy is diverted to the needs of the cancerous cells. If their growth is unchecked, the organism dies and the cancer cells die along with it.

How do cells know when to stop growing? What

makes healthy cells lose the ability to regulate their growth and become cancerous? Over the years, many answers have been given to these questions.

Cancer is often associated with certain chemicals, like tar and soot. According to one explanation, these chemicals produced cancer by "irritation." Another theory held that tiny clumps of embryonic cells, carried over into adult life, suddenly began growing again.

For many years, scientists refused to believe that cancer might be caused by a germ. The only way cancer could be passed from one animal to another was by transplanting the cancer cells themselves. In a new host, the cancer continued to grow just as it had before. This meant that the cause of the cancer was inside the cells themselves.

That was how matters stood in 1911, when a poultry breeder brought a Plymouth Rock hen to the Rockefeller Institute in New York. The hen had a large tumor on her breast. Dr. Peyton Rous, a pathologist at the Institute, examined the tumor cells under a microscope. When he found that they were cancerous, he decided to try an experiment something like the one Beijerinck had performed on tobacco leaves twenty years before.

Dr. Rous ground up the tumor, added water, and passed the mixture through a filter. Then he injected the filtrate into some healthy Plymouth Rock hens. Not all of them were affected by it, but several developed the very same kind of tumor that the filtrate had come from.

Could cancer, like measles and tobacco mosaic disease, be caused by a virus? No one thought so except for Rous. Cancer was a cellular disease, people argued, and its cause must lie inside the cell. In Dr. Rous's experiment, some of the cancerous cells must have passed through the filter and started growing again in the healthy chickens.

These objections were disproved, but Rous's findings were still not accepted. Fowl tumors were one thing, human ones quite another. Since cancer is such a serious disease, it was impossible to repeat Rous's experiments on people. And no one was willing to believe that what was true of chicken tumors could also be true of human ones. For more than twenty years, no further progress was made.

The question of cancer and viruses was reopened in 1932 by Dr. Richard E. Shope, an animal pathologist. Dr. Shope was a rabbit hunter too, and he remembered that wild rabbits sometimes have tumors under the skin of their legs. By performing an experiment very much like Rous's, he was able to show that these rabbit tumors were also caused by a virus. A second virus, the Shope papilloma virus, was shown to cause large, horny growths on the rabbits' necks.

Soon another animal was added to the list. It was known that certain strains of mice were especially likely to develop breast cancer. At first it was thought that this predisposition to cancer was inherited. But in 1936, Dr. John J. Bittner discovered that there was another explanation.

Dr. Bittner found that cancer rarely developed in the offspring of high cancer strain males and low cancer strain females. But when the females came from the high cancer strain and the males from the low one, a high percentage of the baby mice got cancer. The females seemed to be responsible for transmitting it.

Dr. Bittner tried separating the newborn mice from their high cancer strain mothers and having them suckled by females of the low cancer strain. When he did this, the baby mice got almost no cancer at all. The opposite held true too; babies of low cancer strain females had a high incidence of cancer when high cancer strain females suckled them. The cancer-producing agent was in the mothers' milk, and Bittner was able to show that it was a filterable virus.

In the years that followed, evidence linking cancer to viruses continued to mount. Viruses were found to cause cancer in rats, hamsters, dogs, monkeys, and a number of other animals. Being mammals, these animals were more closely related to man than Rous's chickens had been, and many investigators began to suspect that viruses might be responsible for human cancers after all.

Viruses are logical suspects in the search for causes of human cancer. When a cell becomes cancerous, its offspring are cancerous too. For a new trait to be passed on to the next generation, there must be a change in the cell's genetic material. Experiments have shown that viruses are able to bring about just such a change.

The nucleic acid of the virus is the same nucleic acid that genes are made of. Once inside a living cell, a virus can play the role of a gene. Often it does this by taking over the cell's metabolism and forcing it to manufacture new virus particles. But sometimes the virus becomes a permanent part of the cell's genetic material, transforming it from a normal cell to a cancer cell.

Viruses and virus-bearing cells can transform normal cells in tissue culture too. The polyoma virus causes tumors in mice, rats, and hamsters. In a tissue culture of mouse embryo cells, polyoma usually multiplies in the normal way, producing circular regions of dead cells. But once in a while the polyoma virus causes cell transformation. When this happens, the result is a microscopic tumor.

When tissue culture cells are transformed, they lose their contact inhibition. Multiplying in a disorganized way, they pile on top of one another to form a tiny tumor that keeps right on growing. These transformed cells are altered in shape and internal structure, and their genes are abnormal. When cells that have been transformed by the polyoma virus are injected into a healthy mouse, they cause cancer and they stimulate the mouse to produce antibodies that are specific for the polyoma virus.

Although there is no longer any doubt that viruses do cause many cancers, it is difficult to explain just why a certain virus strikes a certain cell at a certain time. Like other viruses, cancer viruses are species specific. A particular virus will produce tumors in some animals but not in others. The adenovirus 12, for example, causes respiratory illness in people, but in baby hamsters it causes cancer. Even in a suitable host a cancer virus may remain latent for many years. Only when it is triggered by chemical irritation, mechanical irritation, or radiation does it spring into action and produce a tumor.

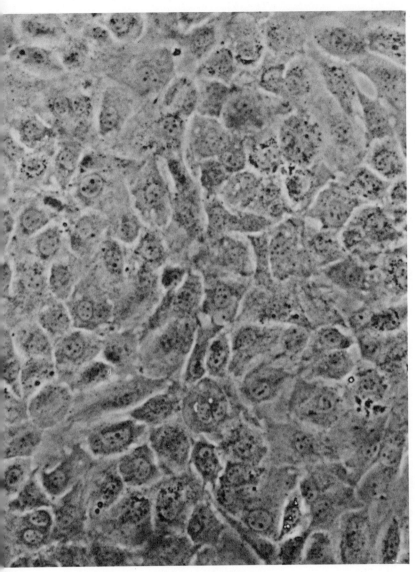

Normal cells growing in tissue culture.

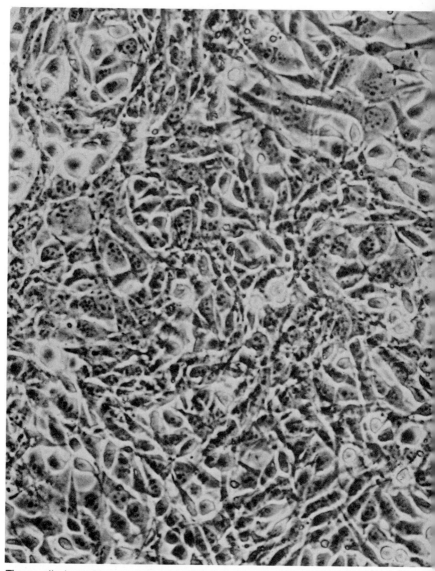

These cells have been transformed by the polyoma virus. They have lost their contact inhibition and changed their size and shape.

Vigorous efforts have been made to find a virus that causes human cancer. Virus particles that appear to be similar to one another have been found in many types of human leukemia. Other viruses have been seen in association with breast cancer and with Burkitt's lymphoma, a tumor of the jaw found mainly in children of tropical Africa. Antibodies against these viruses have been found in many of the cancer patients and even in members of their families. But so far there is no direct proof that the viruses actually cause the cancers with which they are associated.

Many investigators think that such a proof is near at hand. In the words of Dr. Frank J. Rauscher Jr., who heads the virus program of the National Cancer Institute, "We feel we are awfully close." Congress has allocated millions of dollars to the NCI's virus research program. Much of the money is being spent to examine thousands of cancer patients for signs of virus infection and to grow large quantities of the viruses suspected of causing cancer.

If specific viruses can be proven to cause different types of cancer, the chances of prevention would be greatly increased. Already a vaccine has been developed that prevents leukemia in mice. It is not too much to expect that in the future similar vaccines will be able to prevent some human cancers.

16

Correcting Nature's Mistakes

So far, all the viruses in this book have been villains. Bent on their own purposes, they have invaded the sanctuary of the cell and disrupted its normal functioning. But recently scientists have begun to wonder whether viruses, with their unique ability to rewrite a cell's genetic instructions, might also be used to man's advantage.

Sometimes genes are defective. Doctors recognize about 1500 genetic abnormalities, and the average person carries from three to eight of them. Usually these defective genes are masked, and the individuals who carry them don't show their effects. But about 250,000 children are born each year with hereditary defects, 20% of them specifically due to defective genes.

Genetic disease takes many forms. Every gene codes for a specific polypeptide, and a single mistake in this code can be a disaster. Polypeptides are the building blocks from which protein molecules are made. Some proteins are enzymes, substances that govern the body's chemical reactions. A defective enzyme can often mean a defective child.

Phenylketonuria is an enzyme deficiency disease. Children with this disorder are unable to perform one of the chemical reactions essential to normal metabolism, the conversion of phenylalanine to tyrosine. Unless these children are put on a special diet early in life, phenylalanine accumulates in their bodies, resulting in severe mental retardation.

In sickle cell anemia, a disease that affects many black people, the hemoglobin is improperly formed. This can result in growth abnormalities and a generally poor state of health. Sometimes it can even be fatal. Hemophilia, color blindness, and dwarfism are also hereditary diseases. Their symptoms are very different, but all of them can be traced to a genetic abnormality, an inborn error of metabolism.

Someday viruses may be able to rectify these errors. Suppose that DNA could be synthesized to correct a specific genetic defect. If this DNA were attached to the DNA of a virus, infection by that virus could cure the genetic disorder. The virus would multiply, invading the deficient cells and bringing them the information they are lacking.

This kind of genetic engineering has already been observed in the laboratory. In 1949, Dr. Joshua Lederberg and Dr. Norton D. Zinder were experimenting with a bacteria called Salmonella. Bacteria can be given genetic defects similar to the one that causes phenylketonuria. Zinder and Lederberg were working with two strains of Salmonella, each of them unable to produce a different substance essential to its growth. Neither strain could live unless the missing substance was provided in its culture medium.

The investigators mixed the two strains and put them in a medium that lacked both of the key substances. As they expected, the two original strains died out. But in their place a new strain appeared, able to produce both of the missing substances for itself. This new strain was identical to one of the two original ones, except in its ability to manufacture one crucial substance. A genetic defect had been repaired.

Where had this new strain come from? Bacteria have been known to mate, and to combine their genetic material in the process. But in this case only a single trait was transferred. And the bacteria did not have to be in contact for this transfer to take place. The trait could also be transferred in a U-shaped tube, with each strain in its own arm and a bacteria-tight filter between them. Even the addition of a chemical that destroys free DNA did not put a stop to it.

There was only one way that genetic material could pass through a bacteria-tight filter in the presence of a chemical with the power to destroy it, and that was inside a virus. The virus could pass through the filter easily, and its protein coat would serve as protection against the chemical. Sure enough, large numbers of virus particles were found in the bacteria that were contributing the transferred trait.

The investigators were able to show that the bacteria which received the transferred trait carried a hidden virus. In most cases, this virus passed unnoticed from one generation to the next. But once in a while it would spring into action, multiplying inside one bacterium and bursting forth to infect others.

The bacteria that contributed the transferred trait were especially susceptible to infection by this virus. It invaded them in the usual way, using their cellular machinery to reproduce. Occasionally, though, the process went haywire. Of the hundreds of virus particles that were produced, a few got the wrong nucleic acid inside their protein coats. Instead of carrying viral DNA, they carried DNA from the bacteria. When these viruses invaded bacteria of the other strain, they brought them new genes that became a permanent part of their hereditary makeup.

This transfer of hereditary traits by a virus is called transduction. Any trait can be transduced, depending only on the particular DNA that the virus happens to be carrying. In this experiment, the culture medium served to select just those bacteria in which the genetic defect had been eliminated.

How could transduction be used to cure a disease like phenylketonuria? One investigator put it this way: In phenylketonuria, the genetic defect is present in all the cells of the body, but the defective liver cells are the ones that cause the trouble. To cure the patient, the defect in his liver cells would have to be repaired.

Suppose these defective liver cells could be grown in tissue culture and infected with a virus that had multiplied in normal cells. If this virus were capable of transduction, it might supply the liver cells with the gene they needed to produce tyrosine. Since tyrosine is essential to cell growth, a culture medium that did not contain it would serve to select the cells that had acquired the desired trait. These healthy cells could then be returned to the patient's body.

The technical difficulties involved in such a scheme are enormous, but there is reason to hope that someday they can be overcome. In recent years, scientists have synthesized DNA and isolated and synthesized an individual gene. When these techniques can be used to treat genetic disease, they will bring about a new era in medicine.

The authors wish to thank the following persons for their courtesy in permitting in this book the use of the photographs on the pages indicated:

UN photo: page 10.

Dr. W. M. Stanley, Virus Laboratory, University of California: pp. 19, 21, 24.

Dr. Samuel Dales: pp. 26, 29.

Dr. A. K. Kleinschmidt: p. 30.

The Bettmann Archive: p. 38.

Mrs. Hilda Kazaras: p. 41.

WHO photos: pp. 41, 46, 48 (from USIS), 50 (by Homer Page), 84, 89 (by Chevalier), 90, 96.

Dr. Alex J. Steigman; p. 41.

Dr. J. F. Enders: p. 42

National Foundation for Infantile Paralysis: pp. 42 (3).

Dr. A. B. Sabin: p. 49

Merck Sharp and Dohme: pp. 62, 65, 68, 70, 71, 72, 73, 74, 77 (2), 79, 82, 101, 109, 110, 114, 118.

Dr. Maurice Hilleman: p. 66.

Eli Lilly and Company: pp. 76 (2), 80, 81, 82, 104.

Dr. P. J. Imperato, U.S. Public Health Service: pp. 86, 87.

Drs. Lawrence K. Altman and Lewellys K. Barker, N.I.H.: p. 126.

Dr. Renato Dulbecco: pp. 144, 145.

The cover photograph is by courtesy of The State of Alaska, Department of Health and Welfare, and Dr. T. Stephen Jones.

INDEX

About the Authors

Nancy Rosenberg was born in New York City and has lived most of her life in or near the city. She graduated from Bryn Mawr College, Pennsylvania. She has written several picture books for younger readers as well as two previous books on medical subjects: *The Story of Modern Medicine*, which she co-authored with her husband, Dr. Lawrence Rosenberg; and *New Parts for People*, which she co-authored with Dr. Reuven K. Snyderman.

In addition to her career as a writer, Mrs. Rosenberg heads the mathematics department at the Riverdale Country School for Girls. The Rosenbergs and their four children live in Yonkers, New York.

Dr. Louis Z. Cooper is a native of Albany, Georgia, and received his M. D. degree from Yale University. He served in the U. S. Army as a Captain in the Medical Corps, and he is now Associate Professor of Pediatrics and Director of the Rubella Project at New York University Medical Center.

Dr. Cooper has long been interested in prevention, diagnosis, and treatment of infectious diseases, and through his work with rubella research, he became involved with children who were handicapped at birth because their mothers had rubella during pregnancy. As a result of his work with these children, Dr. Cooper now serves on the President's Committee on Mental Retardation and as a Consultant to the U.S. Office of Education, Bureau for the Education of the Handicapped.

The Coopers, who have four children, live in Leonia, New Jersey.